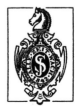

The
Artificial Disc

Edited by
Mario Brock, H. Michael Mayer
and Klaus Weigel

With 51 Figures

Springer-Verlag
Berlin Heidelberg New York
London Paris Tokyo
Hong Kong Barcelona

Professor Dr. Dr. h.c. MARIO BROCK
Dr. H. MICHAEL MAYER
Dr. KLAUS WEIGEL
Universitätsklinikum Steglitz
Neurochirurgische Klinik
Hindenburgdamm 30
1000 Berlin 45, FRG

ISBN-13:978-3-642-75199-8

Library of Congress Cataloging-in-Publication Data. The Artificial disc/edited by Mario Brock, H. Michael Mayer, and Klaus Weigel. p. cm. Includes bibliographical references and index.
ISBN-13:978-3-642-75199-8   e-ISBN-13:978-3-642-75197-4
DOI: 10.1007/978-3-642-75197-4
1. Intervertebral disk prostheses. I. Brock, M. (Mario), 1938– . II. Mayer, H. Michael (Heinz-Michael), 1954– . III. Weigel, Klaus, 1943– . RD755.7.A78 1991 617.3′750592—dc20 90-10417 CIP

This work is subject to copyright. All rights are reserved, whether the whole or part of the material is concerned, specifically the rights of translation, reprinting, reuse of illustrations, recitation, broadcasting, reproduction on microfilms or in other ways, and storage in data banks. Duplication of this publication or parts thereof is only permitted under the provisions of the German Copyright Law of September 9, 1965, in its current version, and a copyright fee must always be paid. Violations fall under the prosecution act of the German Copyright Law.

© Springer-Verlag Berlin Heidelberg 1991
Softcover reprint of the hardcover 1st edition 1991

The use of registered names, trademarks, etc. in this publication does not imply, even in the absence of a specific statement, that such names are exempt from the relevant protective laws and regulations and therefore free for general use.

Product Liability: The publisher can give no guarantee for information about drug dosage and application thereof contained in this book. In every individual case the respective user must check its accuracy by consulting other pharmaceutical literature.

Typesetting: Best-set Typesetter Ltd., Hong Kong
11/3130-543210 – Printed on acid-free paper

Preface

Had we ever guessed the historical importance of this day, had we expected the impressive and touching episode of German history that took place on November 9, 1989, had we dared to hope that a dream three decades old would come true on precisely that day, we would have held our symposium in the immediate vicinity of the Brandenburg Gate! While it is difficult to describe the atmosphere on that evening, when the news suddenly spread that "the wall had opened", it is almost impossible to describe the feeling of fraternity and sense of belonging that overcame everyone, a feeling that had been repressed (but never suppressed) for three decades!

Berlin

M. BROCK
H.M. MAYER
K. WEIGEL

Contents

Introductory Remarks
M. Brock, H.M. Mayer and K. Weigel 1

Functional Anatomy of the Lumbar Spine
R. Louis (With 4 Figures) 3

Implant Materials
H. Stallforth, W. Winkler-Gniewek and M. Ungethüm
(With 4 Figures) 13

Performance of Alloplastic Materials
and Design of an Artificial Disc
H.J. Schmitz, B. Kaden, R.T. Fritz, U. Gross
and G. Fuhrmann (With 9 Figures) 23

Intradiscal Implants in 1989: Concepts and Possibilities
J.A.N. Shepperd (With 4 Figures) 35

Intradiscal Polymerization:
Preliminary Results of Chemical and Biomechanical Studies
A. Garcia, B. Lavignolle, P. Morlier, D. Ducassou
and C. Baquey (With 2 Figures) 39

Intervertebral Implants for Fixation and Disc Replacement
J.A.N. Shepperd (With 6 Figures) 45

Lumbar Interbody Threaded Prostheses
C.D. Ray (With 5 Figures) 53

"Charité Modular": Conception, Experience and Results
H. Zippel (With 3 Figures) 69

Development of a Functional Disc Spacer (Artificial Disc)
C.K. Lee, N.A. Langrana, J.R. Parsons and M.C. Zimmerman
(With 1 Figure) 79

VIII   Contents

The Triazine Carbon Fiber-Reinforced Disc Prosthesis:
Biomechanical and Biological Properties
J. HARMS and H. BÖHM (With 13 Figures) 85

Subject Index 97

List of Contributors

Adresses are given at the beginning of the respective contribution

BAQUEY, C.   39
BÖHM, H.   85
BROCK, M.   1
DUCASSOU, D.   39
FRITZ, R.T.   23
FUHRMANN, G.   23
GARCIA, A.   39
GROSS, U.   23
HARMS, J.   85
KADEN, B.   23
LANGRANA, N.A.   79
LAVIGNOLLE, B.   39
LEE, C.K.   79

LOUIS, R.   3
MAYER, H.M.   1
MORLIER, P.   39
PARSONS, J.R.   79
RAY, C.D.   53
SCHMITZ, H.J.   23
SHEPPERD, J.A.N.   35, 45
STALLFORTH, H.   13
UNGETHÜM, M.   13
WEIGEL, K.   1
WINKLER-GNIEWEK, W.   13
ZIMMERMAN, M.C.   79
ZIPPEL, H.   69

Introductory Remarks

M. BROCK, H.M. MAYER and K. WEIGEL

This volume contains the papers presented at the First International Symposium on The Artificial Disc, held in Berlin Thursday November 9, 1989.

The idea of an artificial disc is not new. As early as 1956, Steenbrugghe et al. [15] referred to an "articular prosthesis" to replace the nucleus pulposus. Several artificial discs have been patented [2–4, 6, 8, 13, 14, 16]. In most of them the disc is either (1) a complex structure composed of felt embedded in plastic, (2) a plastic body containing intercommunicating chambers filled with fluid, or (3) a sandwich-type structure composed of two metallic "end-plates" and one interposed element permitting flexion and rotation [2]. (For an additional review of the pertinent literature see the article by Lee et al. in this volume.) Most of these artificial discs have not withstood – or not even reached – the stage of clinical trial.

The first large series of "replaced discs" was reported by Fernström [5]. His findings, however, were questionable since he occasionally replaced not less than four discs by steel spheres. Obviously, such trials were doomed to failure.

Although artificial joints may be considered an established technology nowadays, and problems related both to materials and to biomechanics have been widely overcome in other parts of the body, the situation is far from solved as concerns the intervertebral disc. The main reasons are:

1. It remains unclear to what extent the intervertebral disc is a joint and/or a bumper.
2. The disc is part of an extremely complicated and not yet fully understood "motion segment," which contains two additional articulations (facets).
3. The size, shape, and function of each individual disc vary both along the spinal column and during life.
4. The disc is a metabolic system, the characteristics of which depend on several factors such as (a) circadian load, (b) topographic peculiarities (both according to the region within a given disc and to its level), and (c) state of degeneration.
5. From the material point of view the disc is highly heterogeneous. Its multiple histological and chemical constituents make the manufacture of a "replica" an almost impossible task.

The Artificial Disc
Ed. by M. Brock, H.M. Mayer and K. Weigel
© Springer-Verlag Berlin Heidelberg 1991

For the neurosurgeon and for other surgeons interested in spinal surgery the above-mentioned facts constitute an irresistible challenge. Since the Department of Neurosurgery at the University Hospital Steglitz in Berlin has had a long-standing interest in the treatment of lumbar disc disease [1, 7, 9-12, 17], it was only natural that the next step should be to gather together the leading groups engaged worldwide in the search for an artificial disc.

The editors of this book hope that the information contained in it may open new roads in this controversial field, much as the opening of the Berlin Wall on the day of our symposium has opened new roads for Europe and for humankind.

References

1. Brock M, Görge HH, Curio G (1984) Intradiscal pressure-volume response: a methodological contribution to chemonucleolysis. J Neurosurg 60:1029–1032
2. Büthner-Janz K, Schellnack K, Helisch H-J, Derr B-G (1986) Bandscheibenprothese. German Patent No DD 239 523 A1
3. Fassio B (1976) Prothèse pour disques intervertébraux. French Patent No 7.637.174, December 3
4. Fassio B, Ginestie JF (1978) Prothèse discale en silicone. Etude expérimentale et premières observations cliniques. Nouv Presse Méd 21: 207
5. Fernström U (1972) Der Bandscheibenersatz mit Erhaltung der Beweglichkeit. In: Erdmann H (Hrsg) Zukunftsaufgaben für die Erforschung und Behandlung von Wirbelsäulenleiden. Hippokrates, Stuttgart, 5: 125–130
6. Frey O, Koch R and Planck H (1987) Gelenkendprothese. European Patent Office. Publication No 0 277 282, October 24
7. Görge HH, Brock M, Curio G, Mayer HM (1986) Surgical findings in 50 cases of failed chemonucleolysis with chymopapain. Surg Neurol 25: 563–567
8. Hoffmann-Daimler S (1972) Bandscheibenprothese. Patent of the Federal Republic of Germany No 2.263.842, December 28
9. Lutze MAW (1986) Intradiskaler Druck/Volumen-Test and Diskographie beim lumbalen Bandscheibenvorfall. Inauguraldissertation, Freie Universität Berlin
10. Mayer HM, Brock M (1988) Percutaneous diskectomy in the treatment of pediatric lumbar disk disease. Surg Neurol 29: 311–314
11. Mayer HM, Brock M (1989) Percutaneous lumbar discectomy. Springer, Berlin Heidelberg New York Tokyo
12. Mayer HM, Lutze M, Wehr M, Kaden B, Brock M (1985) Disc-compliance studies in chemonucleolysis. Alt Spinal Surg 2: 9–11
13. Patil AA (1980) Artificial intervertebral disc. US Patent No 4.309.777, November 13
14. Stubstad JA, Urganiak JR, Kahn P (1972) Prothese zum Ersatz einer beschädigten oder degenerierten Bandscheibe und Verfahren zu ihrer Herstellung. Patent of the Federal Republic of Germany No 22.03.242, January 24
15. van Steenbrugghe HM (1956) Perfectionnements aux prothèses articulaires. French Patent No 1.122.634, May 28
16. Weber BG (1980) Zwischenwirbel-Totalprothese. Patent of the Federal Republic of Germany No 3.023.353, June 21
17. Zamorano L (1985) Komplikationen der Chemonukleolyse in Deutschland. Inauguraldissertation, Freie Universität Berlin

Functional Anatomy of the Lumbar Spine

R. Louis

Knowledge of morphological and functional anatomy allows us to understand the relationship between morphological structures and spinal activity. We will discuss the four main functions of the lumbar spine: statics, stability, neural protection, and biodynamics. Investigation of these functions is necessary in the evaluation of spinal lesions, and their reestablishment should be the primary goal of therapy. The intervertebral disc is involved in all of these functions, and the artificial disc must thus be able to take over all of them.

Lumbar Static Function

The static function of the spine contributes to maintaining the equilibrium of the trunk and head by means of the spinal curvature. The lordotic curvature of the lumbar spine maintains the standing position and allows bipedal locomotion during which the spine lies posterior to the body's center of gravity.

The lumbar curvature with its posterior concavity allows the powerful spinal muscles to counterbalance the anterior forces of gravity. The lumbosacral junction displays a prominent anterior angle known as the lumbosacral angle of the promontory (120°–130°). In the upright position, the vertical line beginning at the center of the polygonal base of the equipoise passes through the cervical vertebral bodies, the body of T12, the posterior surface of the L3 body, and the sacral plate. There is a relation between the lumbar curvature and the position of the hips. Forward hip location corresponds to lumbar kyphosis and backward hip location to hyperlordosis. In our opinion, lumbosacral lordosis is incomplete at birth, undergoing completion after birth by an 18°–23° incurvation of the L5 pars interarticularis during growth. The average angle of the lumbosacral spine between the extreme discs is 45°. In the coronal plane, the lumbar spine is normally straight, except in individuals with pelvic list or scoliosis. An unbalanced lumbar spine exhibits pathological symptoms.

Hôpital de la Conception, 147, Boulevard Baille, 13385 Marseille Cédex 5, France

Regarding static function, placement of one or several artificial discs must avoid creating hyperlordosis with a suprajacent kyphotic compensatory curve due to excessive widening of the intervertebral spaces. Conversely, when there is a kyphotic deformity of the lumbosacral spine resulting from narrowed degenerated discs, artificial discs are able to restore lordosis.

Lumbar Stability

Stability is that quality by which the vertebral structures maintain their cohesion in all physiological positions of the spine. Instability or loss of stability is a pathological process which can lead to the displacement of vertebrae beyond their normal physiological limits.

Our *three-column spine concept* (Fig. 1) is supported by anatomical data from dry European and African skeletons, experiments on fresh cadaver spines, and extensive clinical and surgical experience. It is necessary to consider lumbar stability in both the vertical axis and the transverse plane. *Axial stability* is maintained along a vertical column system; this consists of three columns from C2 to the sacrum. The anterior column is formed by the vertebral bodies and discs, and the two posterior columns by posterior facets and

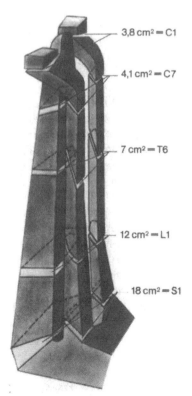

Fig. 1. The three-column concept: The increasing articular surface of the motion segments through the three columns is illustrated

partes interarticulares. This vertical system of columns is reinforced by horizontal struts, pedicles and laminae. Abdominal and spinal muscles add to this stability by acting upon the vertical columns through their insertions on spinous and transverse processes. This three-column structure of the spine, like a three-legged stool, provides the simplest and most efficient system of stability and also protects the neural structures between the columns. *Transverse stability* at the motion segment levels is produced by a coupling of bony buttresses and ligamentous brakes. During flexion, the bony stops are the articular processes and the anterior edge of the end-plates against the upper and lower segment. The ligamentous brakes are all the ligaments located posterior to the nucleus pulposus, i.e., the posterior part of the anulus fibrosus, the posterior longitudinal ligament, the articular capsules, the ligamenta flava, and the inter- and supraspinous ligaments. During extension, the bony stops lie at the angles of a triangle, i.e., the most posterior parts of the articular and spinous processes come into contact with each other and the laminae. The ligamentous brakes involved are situated anterior to the nucleus pulposus. During inclination coupled with rotation, the bony stops are the sagittal part of the facets and the lateral margin of the end-plates. The ligamentous brakes are the intervertebral ligaments opposite the tilt. Another explanation of motion segment stability is our *articular orthogonal theory* (Fig. 2). The three-joint motion segment is characterized by a triangular dis-

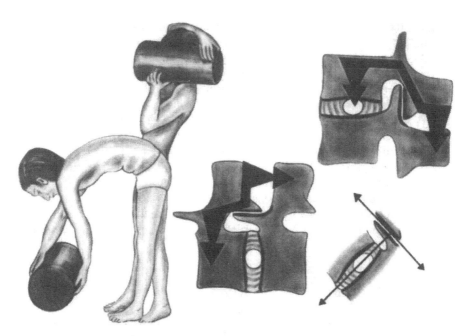

Fig. 2. The articular orthogonal theory. During flexion the facet joints are submitted to compressive forces and the disc to shearing forces. In upright position it is the reverse

position of joints with opposing articular surfaces. At the lumbar region, the posterior joints lie at a 90° angle to the plane of the intervertebral disc. During movement, joint participation differs according to the orientation of the axis of the spine relative to the forces acting upon it. In the vertical position, the forces of gravity and weight-bearing coupled with opposing muscular forces produce a compressive effect on the discs and a shearing effect on the posterior articulations. Conversely, when lifting a weight with the trunk in the horizontal position, the different forces produce essentially compression of the facet joints and a shearing effect on the discs. Consequently, during spinal movement and exertion, the posterior articulations, together with the discs, bear the constraints applied to the vertebrae. Thus, there exists a modulated leverage system involving these different structures. Finally, the zygapophyseal joints should not be considered merely as being involved in the orientation of spinal movement but also as weight-bearing structures subject to the pathological alterations of exertion (sprain and spondylosis). Based on the three-column spinal concept, we state that normal axial spinal growth requires harmonious growth of each column. Consequently, the disturbance of growth leads to scoliosis, kyphosis, or hyperlordosis. The ossification pattern of vertebrae supports our concept. Each column originates from a single primary ossification center. Our stability concept permits an understanding of the constraints to which the spine is subjected: axial pressure along the three columns, pressure on the bony buttresses, the shearing effects on the ligamentous and discal brakes. Depending on the professional activity of patients and their spinal deformity, it is easy to predict the location of age-related arthrosis.

As a result of our stability concept, we proposed, in 1975, a classification of the instability of lesions in order to determine therapeutic indications. Each rupture of a vertical column is given a score of 1; a gap through the anterior column is assessed as 2; and a gap through one posterior column as 1.5. A score equal or superior to 2 indicates an unstable spine.

Artificial disc replacement may produce or intensify spinal instability. After extensive excision of disc material, and especially if superficial anulus layers are thin due to degeneration, instability might result from the disc being submitted to shearing forces when the spine is flexed. On the other hand, when facet cartilage is destroyed by spondylotic lesions, excessive widening of disc interspace by the artificial disc can lead to the loss of contact of facets so that they can no longer play their force-bearing role when the spine is flexed.

Neural Protection

The spine ensures the passage and protection of the neural elements and their annexes through the vertebral canal and intervertebral foramina. The lumbosacral canal has a prismatic shape with an anterior and two posterolateral

Functional Anatomy of the Lumbar Spine

aspects. The anteroposterior diameter of the canal increases from T12–L1 (mean 17.3 mm; range 13–22 mm) to L5–S1 (mean 17.1 mm; range 10–24 mm) and decreases in the direction of the sacral hiatus. The transverse diameter is larger at L1 (19–27 mm; mean 22.9 mm) and L5 (20–35 mm; mean 25.9) than at L3,L4 (22.8 mm) and the sacrum. A narrow lumbar canal frequently has an anteroposterior (AP) diameter of less than 12 mm. The lateral angles of the lumbosacral canal, or lateral recesses, are formed by the pedicles and foraminal inlets. Angles of less than 40° due to osteophytes may result in nerve root compression. The foraminal canals, which are limited by pedicles at their upper and lower ends, have mobile aspects, with discs anteriorly and facet joints posteriorly, liable to compress the spinal nerve by osteophytes and/or disc collapse.

Thus, artificial disc replacement may restore the foramen caliber by intervertebral space widening. Conversely, loosening of the artificial disc may result in narrowing of foramina and/or the vertebral canal with subsequent neural involvement.

Biodynamics

We would like to describe first the joint dynamics and then the neuromeningeal dynamics of the lumbosacral spine.

Joint Dynamics

The five mobile segments of the lumbar spine support its total mobility. Each mobile segment is formed by a set of three joints located at each angle of a triangle and lying in nearly perpendicular planes. These three joints are the intervertebral disc and the two zygapophyseal joints. The discs consist of three parts: the anulus fibrosus, the nucleus pulposus, and the cartilaginous plates. The nucleus pulposus occupies the central core of the anulus fibrosus and, although spherical, does not resemble a solid structure like a ball bearing sealed within the disc, as has often been described. The contents of the nucleus are highly hydrophilic (about 85% water), and the internal resting pressure, ranging from 1.5 kg/cm^2 when recumbent to 10 kg/cm^2 when standing [2], forces the walls of the deepest laminae of the anulus pulposus into their spherical shape. In fact, the nucleus pulposus also displays a loosely packed fibrillar structure continuous with that of the anulus fibrosus, without a clear boundary between the two. The mechanical properties of the disc allow movements of compression when loaded, stretching when distended, rotation about the nucleus, lateral inclination, and translation; however, although an isolated disc allows a wide range of movements between two vertebrae, the presence of the posterior zygapophyseal articulations limits these movements to a spatial sector specific to the lumbosacral spine. The facets of the lumbar vertebrae are inscribed on parabolic curves with a posterior

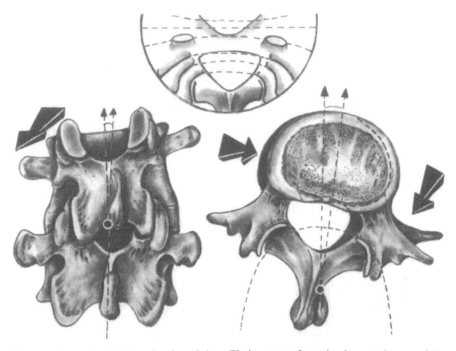

Fig. 3. Dynamics of the lumbar facet joints. Their center of rotation is posterior out of the disc

opening and thus resemble a segment of the groove of a pulley (Fig. 3). This configuration favors flexion-extension movements and is the least adapted to rotational movements.

For the lumbar spine, we stated [1] that the center of rotation for flexion-extension movements was located on the lower end-plate of the disc just below the nucleus pulposus (Fig. 4). Recently, the works of Ogston [37] and Pearcy [4] confirmed this location but confined it to a small area around the point we described. For rotation-inclination, the center of rotation is localized elsewhere, towards the spinous processes, so that the disc undergoes a restricted lateral translation and not a rotational motion around the nucleus pulposus, as generally thought. The mean values for each lumbar motion segment are: flexion-extension, 18°; lateral flexion, 4°; rotation, 3°.

Finally, the three-point piston segment requires a common instability axis of rotation for the disc and the two facet joints in order to avoid further disturbance of the posterior joints. Conversely, when the center of rotation of a spondylotic motion segment projects far from its physiological area, there is an instability with abnormal motion (sliding more than rotating) of the three-joint complex. Surgery (fusion or artificial disc replacement) is not indicated when instability is "microscopic," i.e., when evidenced only by computerized study of flexion-extension centers without any visible abnormal motion on flexion-extension X rays.

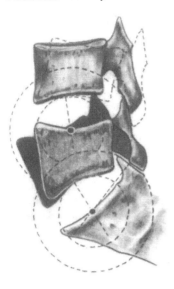

Fig. 4. The center of rotation during flexion-extension is located on the lower end plate under the nucleus pulposus

Neuromeningeal Dynamics

During movements of flexion, the vertebral canal lengthens, as evidenced by the stretching of the posterior surface of the intervertebral discs and the ligamenta flava. Conversely, extension results in a decrease of the length of the vertebral canal. Although the difference in length of the lumbar canal between these two extremes varies among individuals, it is always in the order of several centimeters. Consequently, the intraspinal structures must adapt to these changes in length.

During movements of hyperextension, the dural envelope is characterized by transverse plications, mainly in the region of the interlaminar spaces, and its caliber clearly increases in a transverse and anteroposterior direction. During movements of hyperflexion, the dural envelope lengthens and its surface becomes smooth and stretched, while its caliber decreases in a transverse and anteroposterior direction. Between the positions of extreme hyperextension and hyperflexion, the dura mater stretches and slides along the walls of the vertebral canal. A total variation in length of 50.4 mm of the lumbosacral canal (T12–S1) results in a 39.3 mm change in the length of the lumbosacral dural envelope subjacent to the T12–L1 intervertebral disc (22.5 mm in extension and 16.8 mm in flexion). During extension, the termination of the dural envelope moves as much as 2 mm caudally, whereas hyperflexion causes a mean displacement of 5 mm in a cranial direction. Lengthening and thus stretching of the lumbosacral dural segments increases in the segments closest to the most mobile region, i.e., the L5–S1 region. Accordingly, the dural segment of L1–L2 undergoes a 15% variation in length, compared to 30% at L5–S1. During movements of extension, the lumbosacral nerve roots display regular undulations and distension in the subarachnoid space. In the epidural region up to the outlet of the intervertebral foramen, the tension on each spinal root and nerve relaxes, and the nerves diverge with respect to the pedicles. In the course of hyperflexion, the spinal roots in the cauda equina undergo more complex phenomena, including changes in length and direction and axial displacement.

In short, the L3 nerve root, which retains the same length as in the erect position, constitutes a borderline between the suprajacent roots, which shorten and undulate, and the subjacent roots undergoing progressive stretching in a caudal direction. The nerve roots above L4 are pulled and slide caudally during hyperflexion, whereas the subjacent nerve roots, i.e., L5,S1,S2,S3,S4,S5, and the coccygeal roots, are stretched and slide cranially. The degree of sliding varies according to the level of the spine but can attain 10–12 mm in the intervertebral foramina in the case of roots L5 and S1. The nerve roots above L3 tend to take on a more horizontal position when the spine passes from extension to flexion, whereas the subjacent nerve roots tend to lie more vertically. Subsequently to surgery of the lumbosacral canal, axial mobility of the nerve roots of the cauda equina must be maintained to avoid the painful sequelae of epiduritis. This can be achieved by exercises comprising alternate lifting of the lower limbs while standing. The spinal cord, like the nerve roots, must adapt to the variations in length of the vertebral canal (5–9.7 mm). During forced extension of the spine, the spinal cord displays fine plications near the pia mater, and its caliber increases in relation to its length, which decreases without axial sliding. During forced flexion of the spine, the different segments of the spinal cord, like those of the dura mater, undergo axial displacement towards the most mobile vertebrae of the cervical (C6) and lumbar (L4) regions. Two regions of the spinal cord, the inferior parts of the cervical (C6–T2) and lumbar (L4 to the coccyx) swellings, are submitted to the greatest forces of stretching. These notions of vertebro-medullary dynamics shed light on certain pathological phenomena. Vertebral fracture in hyperflexion may cause neurological lesions without requiring a specific type of bone displacement by elongation analogous to that encountered in lesions of the brachial plexus.

The surgical relevance of these considerations can also be applied to disc displacement. When one or several lumbar discs are collapsed, intervertebral space restoration can reestablish the normal relationship between roots and bony walls of the vertebral anulus foramina. Conversely, the condition of a patient with epiduritis, who has undergone multiple operations, may deteriorate as a result of intervertebral space widening, since adherences pull on the nerve roots.

In conclusion, regarding artificial disc replacement, we have to keep in mind that close attention must be paid to the four functions of the spine in order to allow satisfactory restoration of lumbosacral biodynamics. This is a more ideal aim for spinal surgery than fusion.

References

1. Louis R (1982) Chirurgie du rachis. Springer, Berlin Heidelberg New York Tokyo pp 300, 600 planches anatomiques
2. Nachemson A, Morris JM (1968) Lumbar discometry. Lumbar intradiscal pressure measurements in vivo. The Lancet I: 1140
3. Ogston NG, King GJ, Gertzben SD (1986) Centrade patterns in the lumbar spine. Baseline studies in normal subjects. Spine 11: 591–595
4. Pearcy M, Bogduk N (1988) Instantaneous axes of rotation of the lumbar intervertebral joints. Spine 13(9): 1033–1041

Implant Materials

H. STALLFORTH, W. WINKLER-GNIEWEK and M. UNGETHÜM

Introduction

Based on the knowledge gained from research into corrosion resistance, tissue tolerance, and biomechanics, various materials and material groups have gained acceptance for use in various implant applications (Table 1). They are used as force-transmitting components, such as stabilizing osteosynthesis implants, highly stressed hip joint shafts, or stiffening hip joint sockets. The material or material state to be used in the individual case depends largely on specific requirements.

Every material therefore has its own specific properties, which can be used effectively. High quality, stainless steel is the material mainly used for osteosyntheses because of its excellent cold workability in diverse situations. The cobalt-chromium-molybdenum-based cast alloy has been widely used in endoprosthetics in the joint region due to its excellent wear resistance. Using cobalt-based alloys, above all in the forged version, solved the problem of fatigue fractures in loosened prosthetic shafts. Pure high strength titanium is being used to an increasing extent in place of steel for patients who are allergic to nickel or chromium. Titanium alloys are presently being used in cementless anchoring systems, where the main emphasis is on tissue tolerance (in direct contact with bone) and special mechanical and elastic properties.

Pure metals, such as tantalum, niobium, or even zirconium are important because of their exceptional corrosion properties [2, 3]. Nonetheless, the use of such metals will probably be restricted initially to specific areas of application, such as the substitution of tantalum for silver in neurosurgery, on account of their cost of acquisition and moderate mechanical properties.

These metals can be meaningfully combined with nonmetallic materials, e.g., so as to ensure permanent locomotor function in the joint region. The polyethylene introduced by Charnley [1] for the manufacture of artificial sockets has proved particularly effective in reducing friction. Joint balls made of ceramic materials, e.g., aluminium oxide or zirconium-based, have for the past 10 years contributed to reducing the wear rate of polyethylene.

Aesculap AG, W-7200 Tuttlingen, FRG

Table 1. ISO Standards for Implant Materials

Material	Standards
Alloys	
Fe Cr Ni Mo	ISO 5832/I
Ti	ISO 5832/II
Ti Al V	ISO 5832/III
Co Cr Mo	ISO 5832/IV
Co Cr W Ni	ISO 5832/V
Co Ni Cr Mo	ISO 5832/VI
Co Cr Ni Mo Fe	ISO 5832/VII
Plastics	
PMMA	ISO 5833/1
UHMWPE	ISO 5834/1
	ISO 5834/2
Ceramics	
AI2 O3	ISO 6474

Other plastics are only suitable for special applications, e.g., polyester and polyoxymethylene for slightly stressed joints, such as shoulder and finger joints. The main area of application of polyester is actually in vascular prosthetics, where polytetrafluorethylene and polyurethane are used as alternatives. Silicone rubber, known from plastic surgery, is also used for finger joints.

Anchoring of various prosthetic components in the bone plays a major role. The use of polymethyl methacrylate (PMMA) as a bone cement initially produced spectacular results until complications in the form of loosenings led to disillusionment. This is why attempts are presently being made to dispense with bone cement and to encourage or induce bone growth and clamping to the prosthesis by means of appropriate design and material selection and with the aid of a suitable surface structure and porous of bioactive coating [4].

In the following, the various demands on orthopaedic implant materials will be defined more closely, comparison criteria highlighted, and starting points for future developments mentioned. Experience has shown that no single material exists that can fulfil all expectations simultaneously. Hence, the trend towards composite design has intensified. On the whole, the implant materials must have good tissue tolerance, adequate mechanical properties, and, if necessary, must permit permanent anchoring to bone.

Corrosion Resistance and Tissue Tolerance

Corrosion resistance of all metallic implant materials occurs by virtue of a natural, self-forming protective (passive) layer, which is primarily attributed to the alloying elements chromium and titanium.

Implant Materials

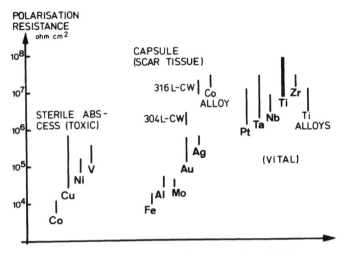

Fig. 1. Corrosion resistance and tissue reaction of different metals and alloys (from Steinemann)

Tissue tolerance is a direct function of corrosion resistance (Fig. 1). Although pure metals, for example, iron and nickel, themselves have slight corrosion resistance in the body, their dissolution is delayed or prevented when they occur as constituents of a passive alloy.

The proven cytotoxicity of individual elements or their known allergenic effect does not have to be feared in general. Nonetheless, individually occurring hypersensitivity reactions in patients to dissolved nickel, cobalt, or even chromium from metallic implant materials is mentioned in the literature, despite a lack of substantiated assessment criteria. Titanium implants, which are known for excellent tissue tolerance, are therefore used for safety reasons, when there is a justified suspicion of an existing allergy.

Mechanical Properties

The mechanical properties of a material are composed of a series of characteristic values, which can be varied within certain limits. These values are determined in tensile tests and ensure that both permanent deformation under foreseeable stress and the risk of fracture are excluded.

In order to ensure a certain safety for the recipient, it is necessary to determine the minimum values of the characteristic mechanical data.

Elasticity, Flexibility, and Rigidity

The implants and thus their materials must meet specifical biomechanical requirements. In order to take over partial or complete function of a bone, an implant must initially have sufficient rigidity. In addition, good fastening or anchoring for efficient force transmission is a prerequisite. Hence, an osteosynthesis implant must be able to keep the bone fragments fixed in place. This is initially achieved when the bone support is applied. Flexibility is desirable when the bone has healed and can assume normal function, for which purpose the rigid implant usually has to be removed.

A prosthetic shaft must prevent bending of the femur when subjected to stress. On the other hand, a certain flexibility would be favorable, so as to transfer part of the load to the bone and therefore encourage a more physiological stress situation. Flexibility is best exploited in the case of slightly stressed joints, e.g., finger joints, where mobility needs to be reestablished.

Flexibility and rigidity are expressions of the elasticity of a material and its ability to reverse under a certain stress, i.e., to expand elastically (Fig. 2). According to Hook, the stress σ, defined as the load per unit area, is proportional to the percentage expansion ε, i.e. to the relative elongation, and the proportional factor is the modulus of elasticity E; $\sigma = E \cdot \varepsilon$; the greater the modulus of elasticity, the more rigid the material.

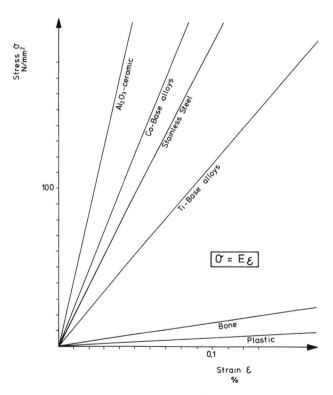

Fig. 2. Hook's rule of the relation between stress (σ) and strain (ε) for different materials and Young's elasticity modulus (E)

Implant Materials

Rigidity can also be influenced via dimensioning. Larger cross sections mean, under the same load, a reduction of stress and accordingly less dislocation.

While stainless steel and cobalt-based alloys have similar rigidity, titanium and its alloys possess about less than half the modulus of elasticity and are therefore considered as being relatively flexible at the same limit of elongation. Although by comparison several plastics, with their low modulus of elasticity, come nearest to bone as stabilizing or reinforcing elements, they can only be used together with a metal core support, metal casing, or by means of fiber reinforcement.

Recently, high tensile, high modulus carbon fibers have been examined on account of their good tissue tolerance. Interesting in this respect, in addition to their low weight, is their radiolucency.

As a rule, ceramic materials possess a high modulus of elasticity. Their behavior under tensile or bending load is unfortunately extremely brittle, i.e., susceptible to fracture; however, they can withstand high compressive load because of their hardness. Zirconium oxide differs from aluminium oxide by its higher bending strength and its modulus of elasticity, which is comparable with that of steel.

Fatigue and Fatigue Strength

Fatigue strength, which is of interest for safe component design, is generally a fraction of the tensile strength. Fatigue strength characterizes the resistance to fracture of metallic materials which are subjected to a constant alternation of load. The dependence of fatigue on the number of alternating cycles is shown in a "WÖHLER diagram" (Fig. 3). The downward sloping lines correspond to the regions of fatigue strength for materials with a finite life. Materials which are loaded according to these values only have a limited life. For a specific stress amplitude, the tolerable number of load cycles is virtually infinite. This special value corresponds to the fatigue strength. In order to avoid fatigue fracture, stressing of the material below this value must be endeavored. This is not always the case where osteosyntheses implants are concerned due to insufficient stabilization, omission of a bone support, or poor healing.

Analysis of prosthetic shaft fractures showed clearly that, in the case of cement-induced loosening, the fatigue limit, especially of casting materials, was brought about as a result of increased stress but above all due to inadequate design or less than optimum positioning. Efforts necessary to increase the fatigue strength of the materials used in the shaft region could thus be noted.

To compare the fatigue behavior of various materials, the fatigue strength under reversed bending stress is determined on smooth test specimens. Since the testing conditions vary to a large extent and the fatigue strength reacts to this very sensitively, the values taken from the literature differ considerably (Fig. 4).

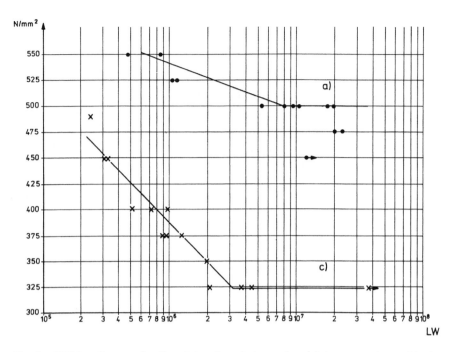

Fig. 3. Wöhler diagram for the state after shot peening (a) in comparison with the polished state of stainless steel (c)

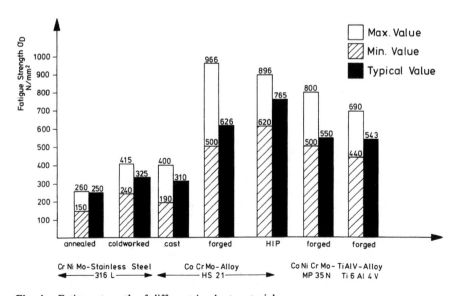

Fig. 4. Fatigue strength of different implant materials

Typical values can be regarded as characteristic of pure materials with the usual structure. Maximum values were achieved by using special surface treatment processes. Shot peening, for example, represents a significant opportunity for further increasing the fatigue strength.

Accordingly, the average fatigue strength of cobalt alloy can be compared with the fatigue strength of steel. By means of effective, subsequent hot formation, e.g., by forging or a special forming process such as the hot isostatic pressing of powder, the fatigue strength is virtually doubled. Hot formation of cobalt cast alloy can give rise to significant problems, such that this material variant for hip joint shafts is only slowly gaining acceptance. Nonetheless, a cobalt-based alloy with a high nickel addition, type MP 35 N, for forged shafts has become popular, since it can be easily shaped. The significance of the forged version of titanium alloy is increasing, since the fatigue strength is exceptional.

Wear Behavior

The actual breakthrough in alloarthroplasty came in 1958 with the introduction of "low-friction arthroplasty" by the English surgeon Charnley [1]. A metal ball, recently also made from ceramic, is articulated against an artificial plastic socket. With a combination of this kind, the wear on the metal or ceramic part is negligible and abrasion on the plastic side is limited.

The cobalt cast alloy has proved suitable for prosthetic arthroplastic balls, since it possesses excellent wear properties. In addition, a very fine surface finish can be achieved. Titanium and its alloys are known for their poor abrasion resistance; even the unproblematic mating with plastic results in metal abrasion so that titanium materials cannot be considered suitable for use as sliding materials.

With ultra-high molecular polyethylene (PE) Charnley [1] discovered, in 1963, the only plastic which up to now has proved suitable in technical and clinical applications. Of particular significance is the fact that PE is biologically and chemically inert and in its ultra-high molecular form has, in addition to good damping properties, exceptional ductility and wear. Nevertheless, as a consequence of cold formation and abrasion, reference can still not be made to an optimum plastic; the majority of substitution attempts, e.g., with teflon, polyester, or admixtures, have failed. Also, the use of polyoxymethylene in the hip joint region failed to produce a convincing result.

Standardization and Development of Implant Materials

A major advance in the clinical application of implants was achieved by standardization of the materials used. Since 1972, a standards Committee TC 150 for surgical implants has existed in the International Standard Organisation, which apart from standards for the form and function of implants also prepares specific material standards. In the summer of this year, a new Standards Committee TC 194 was established for the preparation of standards for the biological testing of medical and dental materials and products. In the same year, a European initiatives as part of the CEN was started.

These activities reflect the requirement both for a standardization of the statutory rules for pharmaceuticals and medical materials and products, in view of the introduction of the European Market in 1992, and for a general obligation for registration. The various Standards committees and endeavoring – through constant revision and introductions – to take into account new developments in the area of orthopaedic implants. With the expansion of the technical possibilities, numerous materials have been listed and classified for use in humans.

New alloys with "memory effect", e.g., based on nickel-titanium (Ni-Ti), promise to provide an especially favorable basis for adaptation to anatomical conditions at the implant site and for the fitting and removal of implants, e.g., for re-operations. They possess the ability, e.g., under the influence of moderate temperature, to take on or revert to their earlier form in situations where the reverse process can also occur. For example, a common indication is the treatment of scoliosis.

Completely new perspectives have been opened by "absorbable" plastics, whose development began with the introduction of suture material. Such plastics, e.g., those which include lactic or glycolic acid, have exceptional strength, so that stabilization of a fracture in the case of slightly stressed bone is already possible today. The absorption of the material makes the removal of the implant – as is common in osteosyntheses – unnecessary.

In conclusion, biological materials should not go unmentioned. With respect to the use of natural tissues, the effects of collagen and other proteins are the subject of intensive research. By removal of the protein and mineral portions of bone, attempts have been made to separate the substances that control bone growth. Although the extraction of these substances seems successful at the present time and their biological effects have been verified, production by gene technology methods still gives rise to numerous unsolved problems.

Thus, the biomechanical compatibility, tissue tolerance, and, if necessary, biological effect of new materials should be verified by various tests prior to the clinical testing. Such tests are indispensible prerequisites, which have to be carried out before any standardization can begin in the research sector. Their registration, as for pharmaceuticals, is imperative.

References

1. Charnley J, Harrey DK (1975) Rate of wear in total hip replacement. Clin Orthop Rel Res 112: 170–178
2. Steinemann SG (1980) Corrosion of surgical implants – in-vivo- and in-vitro-tests. In: Winter GD, Leray JL, de Grot K (eds) Evaluation of biomaterials. Wiley & Sons, New York Chichester
3. Ungethüm M, Winkler-Gniewek W (1984) Metallische Werkstoffe in der Orthopädie und Unfallchirurgie. Thieme, Stuttgart New York
4. Winkler-Gniewek W, Ungethüm M (1984) Extension of the life of implants for osteosynthesis by appropriate shot peening of the surface. In: Niku-Lari (ed) Advances in surface treatments. Pergamon Press, New York

Performance of Alloplastic Materials and Design of an Artificial Disc

H.J. Schmitz[1], B. Kaden[2], R.T. Fritz[3], U. Gross[3] and G. Fuhrmann[4]

Alloplastic materials for hard tissue application, such as metals, metal-ceramic composites, and non-metals, display different chemical and physical properties in the bulk and at the structured surface. Thus, they are differently suited for transmission of tensile, compressive, and shear loads that induce characteristic responses in adjacent tissues and determine individual interfaces. Long-term performance of an artificial disc is guaranteed by interface stability without interfacial soft tissue. Correct matching to biomechanical conditions together with adequate choice of an alloplastic material are prerequisites for successful prosthetic replacement of an intervertebral disc or vertebral body: ridgid – for a fusion, flexible – for a disc endoprosthesis.

Introduction

In general, the original method published by R.B. Cloward in 1958 [3] and modified by Robinson and Smith [2], for intervertebral removal of ruptured cervical discs by an anterior approach has been used. However, homologous bone grafting induces vertebral ankylosis, thus giving rise to overload of neighboring vertebral segments and articulate structures [17, 6]. Methylmethacrylate cement (i.e. Palacos) induces formation of a fibrous, scarred, pseudarthrotic, syndesmotic entity of the vertebrae involved. Theoretical considerations concerning a totally elastodynamic intervertebral disc prosthesis were presented by Edeland [4] in 1981. Bensmann and Salis-Soglio [1] developed an implant made from Ni-Ti memory alloy for partial arthrodesis of the spine. Japanese neurosurgeons Koyama and Handa [10, 11] have already performed implantations of hydroxyapatite in the spines of humans.. Titanium mesh implants and "metal spongiosa" were tested in intervertebral fusions. Further extensive biomechanical, histological, and histomorpho-

---

[1] Klinik für Mund-, Kiefer- und Plastische Gesichtschirurgie, Medizinische Einrichtungen der RWTH, Pauwelsstr., W-5100 Aachen, FRG
[2] Klinik für Neurochirurgie, Klinikum Steglitz, Freie Universität Berlin, Hindenburgdamm 30, 1000 Berlin 45, FRG
[3] Institut für Pathologie, Klinikum Steglitz, Freie Universität Berlin, Hindenburgdamm 30, 1000 Berlin 45, FRG
[4] Bundesanstalt für Materialprüfung (BAM), Unter den Eichen 87, 1000 Berlin 45, FRG

The Artificial Disc
Ed. by M. Brock, H.M. Mayer and K. Weigel
© Springer-Verlag Berlin Heidelberg 1991

metrical research in animals, testing different designs and implant materials, is, however, still needed. Knowledge on hard tissue replacement has increased considerably in recent years. When designing an artificial intervertebral disc prosthesis these experiences should be kept in mind, especially in cervical interbody fusions. Clinical experience in total hip arthroplasty and in oral implantology has revealed that the key to successful performance of implants in bone is mechanical strength of the bone-implant interface. Extensive research in the field of ceramics, polymers, and metals has focused on the development of different porous coatings or rough surfaces in order to improve interfacial load transmission.

Previous studies [5, 9, 12, 13] have already elaborated some prerequisites that are considered to be important for "osseointegration", a term coined by Branemark [2] for long-term anchoring of implants in a bony implantation bed without interference from a soft tissue layer:

1. Porous structure of 50–500 μm in diameter
2. Primary fixation and avoidance of interfacial movements
3. Tight contact of implant and bony bed to enhance ingrowth of bone

Alloplastic materials for hard tissue application are:

Metals: Surgical steel, CoCrMo alloys, titanium, titanium alloys, titanium-ceramic composites

Non-Metals: Glass ceramics, natural or synthetic $CaPO_4$ ceramics (hydroxy-apatite), polymers, carbon-composites

The response to "bioinert" implant materials, such as titanium or titanium alloys, or bioactive bulk materials or coatings, is seen histologically. There is a nearly complete absence of soft tissue seams at implant surfaces, which enhances direct transmission of forces at the interface of incorporated devices. Surface roughness and microporosities create interfaces able to withstand pressure and shear forces. In addition bioactive materials add tensile strength to interfaces, because of physicochemical bone bonding, as occurs for instance with hydroxyapatite, Bioglass, and glass-ceramics (Ceravital). In the past, while searching for and testing new implant materials, push-out or pull-out tests were performed, demonstrating *shear strength* at interfaces. Quantitative figures, however, on *tensile strength* are needed, because there may be mimicry of fixation bonding by surface roughness when performing push-out or pull-out tests. Conclusions concerning interfacial strength from morphological observations alone are scientifically not valid. Strength parameters have to be recorded by biomechanical tests, rather than derived from the close proximity of bone to the implant material. A quantitative biological characterization of the influences of surface structure of alloplastic materials by exact measurement of surface roughness (RT), assessment of ultrastructure by scanning electron microscopy, and standardized tensile testing together with histomorphometry have been performed in recent years. The results have implications for the development of an artificial disc.

Methods

The chemical and physical properties of different alloplastic implant materials and their various surface structures were characterized [8, 16]. Standardized animal experiments were performed in female Chinchilla rabbits. A 3.0 mm burr hole was made sagittally, under constant saline irrigation, into the cancellous bone of the distal femur below the patellar sliding plane. Subsequently the 3.0 mm burr hole was reamed to 3.95 mm using a hollow diamond cylindrical burr. Exactly defined testing cylinders (length, 6.0 mm; diameter, 4.0 mm) with a flattened area (maximum height of 800 μm) parallel to the axis and in accordance with the law of primary bone healing [15], were used, with the flattened area being positioned distally. The standardized cylindrical implants were pressed to fit into these implantation beds. RT was created by sandblasting, which was performed using Al_2O_3 grit as blasting material.

Materials tested were:

1. *Bioactive glass-ceramic (Ceravital)*; RT: 0.06 μm, 10 μm, 28 μm, 52 μm. The implantation period was 84 days.
2. *Pure titanium, (Contimet)*; RT: 5 μm. The implantation periods were 84 and 168 days.
3. *Ti6Al4V alloy*; RTs: 5 μm, 22.7 μm, 36 μm, 47–57 μm; Ti6A14V with wafer-pattern, sandblasted and non-sandblasted specimens; Ti6A14V with slot-pattern, sandblasted and non-sandblasted specimens.
4. *Ti5Al2.5Fe alloy*; RTs: 22 μm, 37–42 μm; Ti5Al2.5Fe with hydroxyapatite (HA) coating; Ti5Al2.5Fe with 33 burr holes, diameter 0.5 mm in the flattened area. The depths of the burr holes were 0.4 mm, 0.8, and 1.2 mm.
5. *Titanium-glass-ceramic composite (HIP-titanium-Ceravital)*; Standardized test specimen with RTs of 5 μm and 28 μm were assessed at periods of 84 and 168 days.
6. *CoCrMo-ASTM-F75 sintered implants* with different mesh sizes of beads; mesh −45 +60 (fine), mesh −60 +80 (middle), and mesh −25 +40 (large). The implantation period was 84 days.
7. *Titanium alloy sintered implants* with different mesh sizes of beads; mesh 30–35 (fine), mesh 20–25 (middle), and mesh 18–20 (large). Implantation periods of the different materials were 84 days, 168 days, or up to 1 year.
8. *Polymethylmethacrylate (PMMA) cement (PALACOS)*; implanted within a hollow tubing (test samples 6.0 × 4.0 mm) with flattened area parallel to the axis (maximum height, 800 μm); implanted for 84 days.

9. *Polytetrafluorethylene (PTFE) (PROPLAST)*; within hollow Ti6Al4V tubing as standardized test samples and with the bone having access to the PTFE material at the flattened area; implanted for 84 days.

After these intervals the implant specimens were removed together with the adjacent bone. Samples were prepared for tensile and histomorphometrical and histological analyses. For representative histomorphological evaluation, undecalcified sections were prepared from each implanted specimen by use of a sawing microtome. Sections were stained with Giemsa solution or within on Kossa'-Fuchsin. Quantitative histomorphometrical analysis was performed by recording percentages of bone, osteoid, chondroid, and soft tissue at the implant surfaces. Tensile testing was performed as described previously [8].

Results

Bioactive Glass-Ceramic. After 84 days bioactive glass-ceramic (Ceravital) showed a tensile strength of about 1 N/mm^2. The tensile strength relating to different RTs are given in Fig. 1. Histomorphometrical analysis revealed more than 80% bone at the implant surface and almost no osteoid and no chondroid tissue.

Pure Titanium (Contimet). After 84 and 168 days, this smooth surfaced material (RT 5 µm), exhibited no bone bonding or tensile strength. Histomorphometrically, nearly 100% of the surface was covered by a very small soft tissue seam. In some areas contact of bone to the titanium surface was observed.

Ti6Al4V Alloy. The same result was obtained for Ti6Al4V alloy, at 84 and 168 days, when its surface was smooth (RT 5 µm) as for pure titanium. Increased

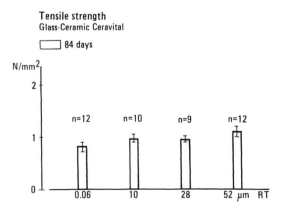

Fig. 1. Tensile strength ± SEM of Ceravital with different surface roughnesses (*RT*). *n* = number of samples

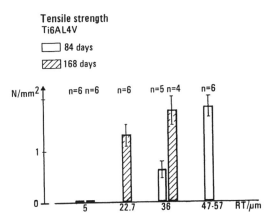

Fig. 2. Tensile strength of Ti6Al4V ± SEM as a function of surface roughness (RT)

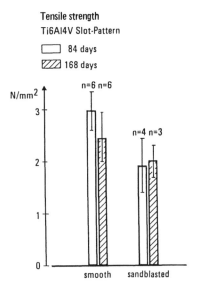

Fig. 3. Tensile strength ± SEM of Ti6Al4V with slot-pattern

RT by sandblasting induced a tensile strength of the magnitude of $1-2 \, N/mm^2$ (Fig. 2). The Ti6Al4V-slot pattern exhibited the highest values of tensile strength after 84 days. Longer implantation time and additional sandblasting did not result in increased tensile strength. The reason for this rather detrimental and unexpected result was given by histomorphometrical analysis showing that slots with a diameter of 0.5 mm were covered by a very thin layer of mineralized bone only, whereas almost all of the total volume of most other slots was replaced by bone marrow, indicating the absence of a suitable pattern for mechanical interlocking with bone (Figs. 3, 4). The Ti6Al4V-wafer pattern at the flattened

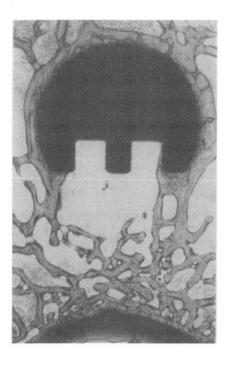

Fig. 4. The histomorphology of Ti6Al4V with slot-pattern

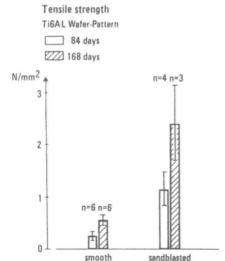

Fig. 5. Tensile strength ± SEM of Ti6Al4V with wafer-pattern

surface displayed no convincing advantage when smooth; sandblasting, however, increased tensile strength to about 1 N/mm^2 after 84 days and above 2 N/mm^2 at 168 days (Figs. 5, 6).

Ti5Al2.5Fe Alloy. The results obtained for different sandblasted specimens of Ti5Al2.5Fe alloy were similar to those for surfaced Ti6Al4V specimens.

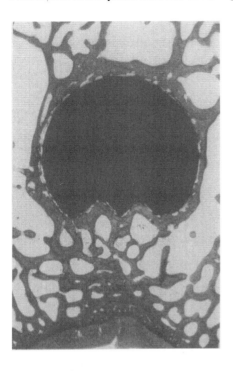

Fig. 6. The histomorphology of Ti6Al4V with wafer-pattern

The data for tensile strength are given in Fig. 7. Different surface patterns influenced the retentive potential for ingrowth of bone. Ti5Al2.5Fe, with 33 burr holes with a diameter of 0.5 mm and different depths, increased the tensile strength of the interface to 2.2–2.8 N/mm^2 after 84 days and more than 3 N/mm^2 after 168 days (Fig. 7). Histomorphometrical and scanning electron microscopical analyses showed complete bone mineralization of the 0.5 mm deep burr holes; in deeper holes (0.8 and 1.2 mm) there was no mineralization at the bottom of the holes. Ti5Al2.5Fe with HA coating was nearly as strong as non-HA coated but rough surfaced titanium alloy implants (Fig. 7). In some specimens detachment of the HA coating from the bulk material was observed, demonstrating the current problems of coating technology.

Titanium-Glass-Ceramic Composite (HIP-titanium-Ceravital). Standardized test specimens with RTs of 5 μm and 28 μm were assessed at periods of 84 and 168 days. Tensile strength amounted to 1.2 ± 0.41 N/mm^2 after 84 days and 1.3 ± 0.34 N/mm^2 after 168 days. Histomorphometry showed favorable behavior, similar to glass-ceramic (Ceravital). Mechanical properties, however, suggested its use as a coating material on titanium alloy cores.

Cobalt-Chromium Implants with Multilayers of Beads. Sintered implants, with porous coatings of CoCrMo-ASTM F-75 beads with different mesh sizes, also exhibited quite promising tensile strength, amounting to about 3 or in the

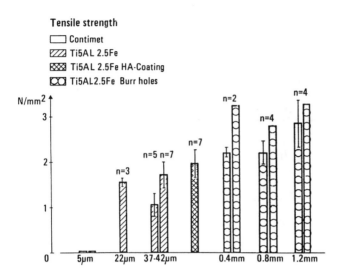

Fig. 7. Tensile strength ± SEM of differently surfaced Ti5Al2.5Fe samples

finest mesh even above 4 N/mm^2 (Fig. 8). Histomorphometrical analysis of porous coated CoCrMo-ASTM F-75 implants revealed a diameter of 0.33 mm for fine and 0.58 and 0.89 mm for the larger beads. Mineralized bone was detectable up to a distance of 1–1.5 mm from the surface coating. In the base of the coating layers only blood cells, soft tissue, and tissue fluid were found; thus, more than two to three layers are not recommended.

Titanium Alloy Monolayer Sintered Implants. Ti6Al4V specimens with a monolayer of different mesh sizes of titanium beads (mesh 30–35 = fine, mesh 20–25 = middle, and mesh 18–20 = large), developed tensile strength in the order of 3–4 N/mm^2 after 84 days. There were no statistically significant differences between the different pore sizes tested (Table 1). A tendency towards slightly higher strength in monolayer Ti6Al4V specimens after 84 days was noted. Histomorphometry revealed well-mineralized bony tissue within the pores (Fig. 9). Extended implantation time (1 year) resulted in quite notable further increases in tensile strength, up to 6–7 N/mm^2, which is close to the proper strength of trabecular bone itself. Scanning electron microscopic pictures indicated a lamellar structure of trabeculae anchoring in the porous surface. No nonvital tissue or cells were noted in the depths of these madreporic monolayer surface structures.

PMMA Cement (Palacos). These were implanted as 6.0 × 4.0 mm test samples with a flattened area 800 µm parallel to the axis. Tensile forces recorded in the standardized rabbit model were in the order of 0.1–0.2 N/mm^2, i.e. close to zero.

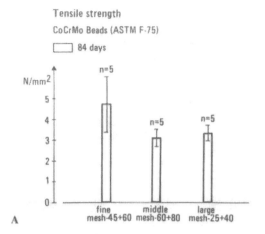

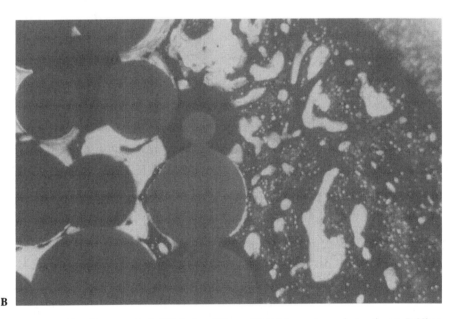

Fig. 8. A Tensile strength ± SEM of multilayer CoCrMo madreporic specimen. **B** Histomorphology of multilayer CoCrMo madreporic-surfaced implants. Ingrowth of mature bone into superficial layers only. Tissue fluids and potentially nonvital material accumulating in depth of pores

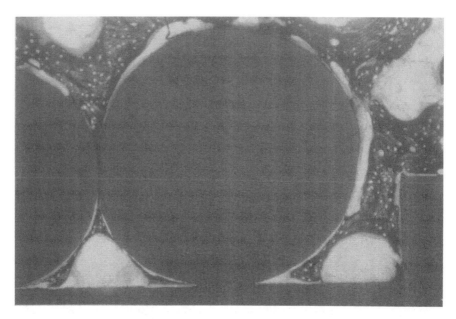

Fig. 9. Monolayer Ti6Al4V madreporic specimen, 168 days

Table 1. Tensile strength of monolayer beads surfaced with Ti6Al4V after implantation periods of 84 days or 1 year

Material	Mesh	Tensile strength (N/mm^2)	n
Ti6Al4V 4.0 × 6.0 mm	30–35	5.18 ± 1.35	3
(porous coated cylinders)	20–25	3.63 ± 0.37	4
84 days	18–20	5.25 ± 0.57	4
Ti6Al4V 4.0 × 6.0 mm	30–35	6.34 ± 0.36	4
(porous coated cylinders)	20–25	6.76 ± 0.49	4
1 year	18–20	5.71 ± 0.45	4

PTFE (Proplast). These standardized test samples exhibited low tensile forces due to ingrowth of bone. Mechanical properties, however, do not recommend the porous material as a load-bearing, hard tissue substitute.

Discussion

Standardized application of tensile testing and additional histomorphometrical analysis in parallel prospective experiments are essential prerequisites for further refinement and development of surface treated alloplastic implants.

Interfacial strength of bioactive glass-ceramic (e.g., Ceravital) is nearly unaffected by sandblasting and without an increase in the magnitude of bone bonding. Scanning electron microscopy reveals shell-like structures which do not offer retentive patterns for anchoring of fibrils or osteocytes. Smooth surfaced titanium implants (RT <10 μm) have no interfaces to withstand tensile forces. Creation of retention patterns by sandblasting of Ti6Al4V or Ti5Al2.5Fe alloys enabled the development of interfacial mechanical bonding between implants and surrounding mineralized hard tissue because of interlocking or interdigitation of fibrils and osteocytes with protruding or intruding surface structures. The magnitude of tensile strength which might be obtained in rough surfaced titanium alloy is of the same order as in bioactive specimens or even higher. Experiments with different degrees of surface roughness show one- or twofold increases in tensile strength. HIP sintered, secondarily porous surfaces of metal-ceramic composites exhibited tensile strengths of comparable magnitudes. Experiments with slot-pattern implants, however, revealed the complexity of the problem. Geometrical factors seem to influence ingrowth of bone; stress-shielding phenomena may also account for the absence or incomplete ingrowth of bone into certain kinds of slots. The required optimum surface should have structures for anchoring of tissue at micrometer scale level to increase local shear phenomena without inducing stress shielding. Depending on its chemical and physical properties, it is differently suited for transmission of tensile, compressive, and shear loads inducing characteristic responses in adjacent tissues and thus determining individual interfaces. Long-term performance of an artificial disc is guaranteed by interface stability without interfacial soft tissue. Correct matching to biomechanical conditions and adequate choice of alloplastic material, are prerequisite factors for successful prosthetic replacement of an intervertebral disc or vertebral body, rigid – for a fusion, flexible – for a disc endoprosthesis.

Acknowledgements. This study was supported by the Ministry for Research and Technology, Bonn, FRG, Grant 01 ZQ 110, E. Leitz Wetzlar, 6330 Wetzlar, FRG, and Mecron, 1000 Berlin 49, FRG.

References

1. Bensmann G, Salis-Soglio GV (1984) Distanzstück aus Nickel/Titan für partielle Wirbelsäulenversteifungen. Technische Mitteilungen Krupp Forschungsbericht, Bd. 42: Heft 1
2. Branemark P-I, Hansson B-O, Adell R, Breine U, Lindström J, Hallen Q, Ohman A (1977) Osseointegrated implants in the treatment of the endentulous jaw. Scan J Plast Reconstr Surg (Suppl 11) 16: 1–131
3. Cloward RB (1958) The anterior approach for removal of ruptured cervical discs. J Neurosurg 15: 602–617
4. Edeland HG (1981) Suggestions for a total elasto-dynamic intervertebral disc-prosthesis. Biomat 9: 65–72

34 H.J. SCHMITZ et al.: Performance of Alloplastic Materials

5. Engh CA, Bobyn JD (1985) Biological fixation in total HIP arthroplasty. SLACK Inc., 6900 Grove road. Thorofare NJ 08086
6. Goel VK, Clark CR, McGowan D, Goyal S (1984) An in-vitro study of the kinematics of the normal, injured and stabilized cervical spine. J Biomech 17: 363–376
7. Gross UM, Strunz V (1977) Surface staining of sawed sections of undecalcified bone containing alloplastic implants. Stain Technol 52: 217–219
8. Gross UM, Roggendorf W, Schmitz H-J, Strunz V (1987) Biomechanical and morphometrical testing methods for porous and surface reactive biomaterials. In: Lemons JE (ed) Quantitative characterization and performânce of porous implants for hard tissue applications. American Society for Testing and Materials, pp 330–346, ASTM STP 953, Philadelphia
9. Hulbert SF, Young SA, Mathews RS, Klawitter JJ, Talbert CB, Stelling FH (1970) Potential of ceramic materials as permanently implantable skeletal prostheses. J Biomed Mater Res 4: 433–456
10. Koyama T, Handa J (1985) Cervical laminoplasty using apatite beads as implants. Surg Neurol 24: 663–667
11. Koyama T, Handa J (1986) Porous Hydroxyapatite ceramics for use in neurosurgical practice. Surg Neurol 25: 71–73
12. Pilliar RM, Cameron HO, Szivek J, Binnington AG, MacNab I (1979) Bone ingrowth and stress-shielding with a porous surface coated fracture fixation plate. J Biomed Mater Res 13: 799–810
13. Pilliar RM, Cameron HO, Welsh RP, Binnington AG (1981) Radiographic and morphologic studies of load-bearing porous-surfaced structured implants. Clin Orthop 156: 249–256
14. Robinson RA, Smith GW (1955) Anterolateral disc removal and interbody fusion for cervical disc syndrome. Bull Johns Hopkins Hosp 96: 223–224
15. Schenk RK, Willenegger HR (1977) Zur Histologie der primären Knochenheilung. Unfallheilkunde 80: 155–160
16. Schmitz H-J (1988) Wirkung chemischer und physikalischer Faktoren alloplastischer Implantatmaterialien auf Gewebe und Biomechanik in tierexperimentellen Modellen. Dissertation, FU Berlin
17. Whitehill R, Barry J (1985) The evolution of stability in cervical spinal constructs using either autogenous bone graft or methylmethacrylate cement. Spine 10: 32–41

Intradiscal Implants in 1989: Concepts and Possibilities

J.A.N. Shepperd

The forms of back pain other than sciatica continue to pose an unresolved challenge to surgeons. For the most part we must admit a profound ignorance as to its cause and acknowledge that surgery for this complaint is quite often a failure, even to the extent of worsening a patient's condition. Dysfunction of a disc may be perceived as the cause, but our understanding of disc dynamics is limited. Before contemplating prosthetic substitutes or other intradiscal devices, the inner world of the disc has to be considered.

We have studied sagittal half spines in 84 segments to observe the internal mechanics and aging changes which occur. Fresh postmortem specimens were collected and prepared by freezing and surfacing the sagittal interface. The specimens were mounted in a frame and subjected to compression and traction. Following this, loaded flexion and extension were studied, recorded by X-ray, photography, and video. The specimens ranged from neonates to the elderly and a pattern of aging changes emerged. In early life, the nucleus and inner annulus are tethered by collagen fibers to end plate cartilage and bone (Fig. 1). End plate pressure is borne by the annulus and nucleus in varying ratios depending on the hydration of the nucleus. The hydrostatic pressure of the nucleus is maintained by the collagen matrix of its own structure, like a sponge. It is, therefore, not normally liable to explode, and the act of "nucleotomy" has little effect on a normal young disc.

Movement of the spine produces characteristic dynamics of the nucleus. In flexion the nucleus moves posterior, and in extension it moves anterior (Fig. 2). This consistent feature means that the motion segment joint is polycentric. The range of movement varied among individual specimens, whose tissues had varying physical properties. It is also greater when the nucleus is more hydrated. This dynamic arrangement is likely to account for inevitable aging changes, which should not be labelled as pathological (Fig. 3). In early adult life, fault lines appear at the boundary between the nucleus and end plate cartilage, seen as a horizontal H configuration on discography. The collagen component of the nucleus increases with age, possibly as a repair attempt from the continual sheer forces which arise within its structure. Disc

---

Hastings Orthopaedic Centre, Royal East Sussex Hospital, Hastings,
East Sussex TN 34 1 ER, U.K.

The Artificial Disc
Ed. by M. Brock, H.M. Mayer and K. Weigel
© Springer-Verlag Berlin Heidelberg 1991

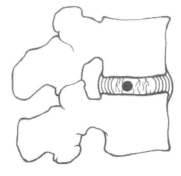

Fig. 1. In early life the nucleus and inner annulus are tethered by collagen fibers to end plate cartilage and bone respectively. Hydration of the nucleus determines the ratio of load born between annulus and nucleus

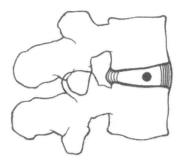

Fig. 2. Movement of the spine produces characteristic internal dynamics of the nucleus such that in flexion the nucleus moves posterior and in extension it moves anterior, making the joint polycentric

chondrocytes are concentrated at the end plate cartilage and inner annulus, but it is not clear whether these cells are also responsible for collagen production. Changes gradually extend towards the disc periphery. Buckling and disruption of the inner posterior annulus are commonly seen by the midthirties, associated with more obvious horizontal fissuring at the earlier fault lines. Increase in anteroposterior movement of the nucleus may occur with less control, setting the scene for patterns of disc herniation. Such herniation may not result in symptoms for the patient, depending perhaps upon irritation of posterior longitudinal ligament and/or theca, and/or nerve roots. Symptoms are almost always episodic, and healing followed by long remission is the rule.

Patterns of late disc disruption include extension of the fault line into a vertical anterior fissure, which mirrors the line of the facet joint and corresponds to a lowering of the center of movement of the motion segment from the nucleus to a point within the substance of the lower vertebra. This change warps the facet joint articulation and may lead to disruption and degenerative spondylolisthesis. Nerve roots may be affected, particularly in the lateral recess, by soft tissue disc herniations, inflammatory episodes from the lateral expansion of the posterior longitudinal ligament, inflammatory episodes from the facet joint, or loss of disc height producing bunching of the soft tissues and cephalad advance of the superior facet.

All these changes frequently arise without the individual suffering any symptoms at all. Appropriate selection of patients depends on provocative

Intradiscal Implants in 1989: Concepts and Possibilities

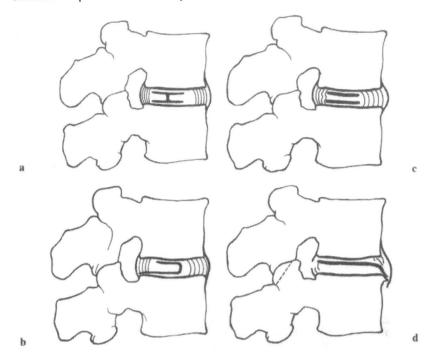

Fig. 3a–d. Aging changes. **a** By early adult life fault lines appear at the boundary between the nucleus and the end plate cartilage, yielding a characteristic horizontal H configuration on discography. **b** The fault lines develop with aging to become horizontal fissures which may then extend posteriorly to the longitudinal ligament **c** or extend into a vertical anterior fissure **d**. The theoretical end stage of fibrous or bony ankylosis only occurs rarely

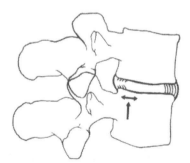

Fig. 4. Loss of nucleus support provokes grinding and thereby destruction of the posterior annulus

testing, as in spinal probing, in order to confirm a pain source and reversibility.

Intradiscal therapies for symptomatic patients range from the use of anti-inflammatory steroids, chemical disruption of the proteoglycans matrix, excision of varying quantities of nucleus material, laser attack on the nuclear material, and fixation of the motion segment. Loss of nuclear support leads to grinding and thereby attenuation of the posterior annulus (Fig. 4).

Thus there are significant disadvantages to all the methods at the present time, and they do not restore normal function. Disc ablation in varying degrees can only result in functional change affecting either disc height and thereby the lateral recess, or segmental instability with irritation of the posterior longitudinal ligament. Fusion considerably alters the mechanics of adjacent segments and may thereby generate a domino effect. Restoration of "normal" disc height and function artificially is an ideal objective in theory, although wear debris and deterioration of the device could lead to disastrous failures.

Intradiscal Polymerization:
Preliminary Results of Chemical
and Biomechanical Studies

A. Garcia[1], B. Lavignolle[2], P. Morlier[3], D. Ducassou[1]
and C. Baquey[1]

Introduction

The purpose of the present study is to provide a prosthetic replacement for damaged intervertebral discs using a posterolateral percutaneous approach.

Historically, two methods have been followed in the development of disc prostheses. The first, for which the Link prosthesis provides an excellent example, is to replace the whole disc and adjacent end plates. The second is to replace only a part of the damaged disc, especially the nucleus. This method became conceivable when chemonucleolysis and, later, nucleotomy began to be used.

Some investigators have tried to maintain the space between the vertebral bodies without any means of restoring the elastic properties of the inter-vertebral joints. An example is given by the approach used by Shepperd [4] in Great Britain. Nonetheless, this type of prosthesis has advantages over spinal fusion, in which homografted bone is employed.

Several authors [1, 2, 3] have also envisaged a prosthesis that restores the main functions of the disc, i.e., maintains the original thickness of the disc, its shock absorbing properties, and the natural bending of the joint. This approach was chosen in the present study. The main goals were:

1. Replacement of a damaged nucleus with a suitable material after nucleotomy using a posterolateral percutaneous approach
2. Preservation of the anulus outer layers to hold the prosthesis in place
3. Selection of a material able to replace the nucleus with regard to hard-ness, elasticity, and resistance to compression
4. Prevention of secondary herniation

Material and Methods

Material Selection

Polyurethanes, which are characterized by compressibility, tensility, resist-ance to shear, and impact strength of the same order as a normal disc, were

---

[1] 9, Allee Boissiére, 33980 Audenge, France
[2] Anatomy and Biomechanical Department Bordeaux II, France
[3] Department of Civil Engineering, Faculté des Sciences, Bordeaux I, France

The Artificial Disc
Ed. by M. Brock, H.M. Mayer and K. Weigel
© Springer-Verlag Berlin Heidelberg 1991

40 A. GARCIA et al.

chosen. They are physiologically inert, nonirritating and nonallergenic and thus may be used in orthopaedic surgery. Moreover, they can be formed in place without the application of heat or pressure, completely filling irregular cavities in which the prepolymer materials are placed.

Polyurethane elastomers are formed by chemical reactions between diisocyanates, short polyols, long polyols, and a polymerization catalyst:

Diisocyanates
or   + Long Polyols + Short Polyols → Polyurethane
Triiosocyanates

The mechanical characteristics of polyurethanes are determined by: (a) the number of isocyanate groups (triisocynates give cross-linked networks of polymer molecules), (b) the polyol's number of hydroxyl groups, (c) the polyol's molecular weight, and (d) the ratio of short to long polyols.

The characteristics sought were based on the disc physiological data summarized in Table 1. To make samples, the prepolymer was cast into matrices 40 mm high and 25 mm in diameter and subsequently examined using a computer-controlled hydraulic testing machine (2000 daN max.). First, the prepolymer mixture was chosen on the basis of its gelation rate (30 min at 37°C). Second, the mechanical properties of the selected polymer were tested by increasing the strain until the breaking point (at 25°C) was reached. Third, the PU 4 of the selected polymer was tested with hysteresis strains between 2 Mpa and 6 Mpa, each sample being subjected to ten cycles (Fig. 1).

Behavior of the Selected Polymer Polymerized in the Nuclear Cavity Under Increasing Strain

Pig Intervertebral Joints. Initially, trials were made on fresh pig intervertebral joints. After removal of the vertebral arch and paravertebral soft tissues, the spines were dissected into segments consisting of two vertebrae and the intervening disc. In some cases four joints from the same spinal column were available for testing. Eight joints in all were tested. Each half vertebral body was fixed in a small, polymethacrylate cement cylinder, each vertebra having about three quarters of its vertebral body embedded. Care was taken during mounting to ensure that the plane midway through the intervertebral disc was parallel to the end plates of the containers holding the upper and lower vertebrae. A computer-controlled hydraulic machine was again used to test

Table 1. Requirements for design of a disc prosthesis

Axial compression resistance	Young's module	Polymerization temperature	Gelation rate
>3 MPa	<70 MPa	37°C	30 min

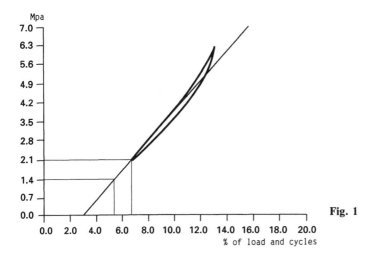

Fig. 1

the joint. For the same spinal column we tested: two normal joints; one joint filled with the selected polymer in place of the extracted nucleus; and one joint with extracted nucleus (using nucleotomy forceps) only.

For each series, an axial compressive strain increasing from 0 MPa to 2.4 MPa and then back to 0 MPa was applied. In each case, the return to baseline was controlled. Following the trial, each joint was compressed until the breaking point. The behavior of the disc and the polymer-filled joint was subsequently examined by axial section.

Human Intervertebral Joints. We are currently beginning the same tests with human cadaveric joints.

Results

Polymer Selection

The mechanical characteristics of the polyurethane samples are summarized in Table 2. The Young's modules and breaking strains increased in accordance with short and long polyol ratios. Samples PU3 and PU4 resisted all strains tested with the available machine (max. 2000 daN). Sample PU4 was selected on the basis of the data presented above.

Table 2. Mechanical characteristics of the polyurethane samples

Sample number	PU 1	PU 2	PU 3	PU 4
Young's module	4.8 Mpa	11.5 Mpa	12.1 Mpa	24.8 Mpa
Breaking strain	4.9 Mpa	11.8 Mpa	Not attained	

PU4 Behavior Under Cyclic Strain

After ten cycles, the hysteresis measurements revealed no significance spreading for this polymer. Furthermore, the Young's modules remained compatible with the physiological data (Fig. 1 and Table 3).

PU4's Behavior Inside a Pig Intervertebral Joint

The polymerized disc showed a behavior similar to that of a normal one (Fig. 2). By contrast, the joint with an extracted nucleus only showed considerable hysteresis with a longer comeback range; this was an unstable joint. The breaking strain results are summarized in Table 4. Young's module value of the polymerized disc is between those of the normal and nucleotomized discs. While the breaking strains of normal discs are determined by the disc itself, the breaking strain of the vertebral joint containing a polymerized disc becomes determined by the end plates (compare value in column three with that of the nucleotomized disc). It is also important to note that the polymer was still in place after experimentation.

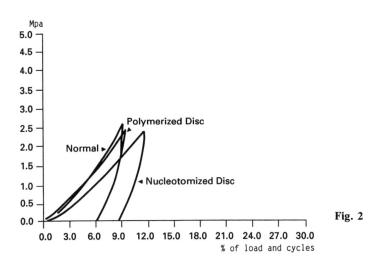

Fig. 2

Table 3. Measurement of Young's module for polyurethane (PU) 4

	PU 4.1	*PU 4.2*	*PU 4.3*
Young's modules	24.07 MPa	23.7 MPa	24.08 MPa

Intradiscal Polymerization

Table 4. Breaking strain results

	Normal disc 1	Normal disc 2	Polymerized disc	Nucleotomized disc
Young's module	18.65 MPa	17.50 MPa	15.50 MPa	12.5 MPa
Breaking strain	4.81 MPa	4.79 MPa	6.30 MPa	6.39 MPa

Table 5. Comparison of complete and partial disc prostheses

	Complete prosthesis	Partial prosthesis
Insertion		
Approach	Ventral	Posterolateral
Duration	60–120 min	30–40 min
Surgical risk	High	Low
Stress	High	Low
Removal	Difficult	Easy
Shock absorption	+	+++
Space maintenance	+++	++

Conclusion

Preliminary results of this study suggest that it may be possible, using polymerization into the disc, to artificially restore the physiological properties of the vertebral joint after nucleotomy. The posterolateral percutaneous approach has advantages over the ventral one; major features comparing complete and partial disc prostheses are summarized in Table 5.

Future work on the method reported here will address the necessity of injecting the prepolymer into a small plastic bag to avoid disc reherniation and will examine ways to permanently anchor the prosthesis in place.

References

1. Froning E (1974) Intervertebral disc prosthesis. U.S.P.
2. Mandarino MP (1962) Methods and materials for orthopedic surgery U.S.P.
3. Ray CD (1988)
4. Shepperd JAN (1987) Posthepatic disc U.S.

Intervertebral Implants for Fixation and Disc Replacement

J.A.N. Shepperd

This chapter covers the Hastings approach and surgical background in relation to intradiscal implants for both immobilisation and prosthetic substitution of the disc. This Centre is committed to the principle of minimal intervention surgery where possible. Elaborate posterior operations may produce permanent deficiency of the posterior musculature, and anterior surgery is potentially hazardous. Two surgical approaches are employed, namely blind percutaneous postero-lateral access and postero-medial minimal intervention fenestration (MIF) (Fig. 1). These will now be described.

Blind Percutaneous Access

Using the conventional X-ray controlled 45° postero-lateral approach, it has been established by cadaver studies that an access tube of 1-cm diameter may be safely introduced in the majority of cases provided the following strict criteria are met: (a) a blunt edged introductory probe reduces the risk of transfixing soft tissues, (b) the entry point to the disc is very precisely at the posterior border of the vertebral body, and in line with the outer border of the pedicle in the anterior-posterior view (it is also at the middle or lower half of the disc), and (c) ascending rigid coaxial tubes must have a close-fitting leading age with a bevel of no more than 2.5 mm. The method requires previous experience and should under no circumstances be employed without instruction. Nevertheless, it is outside the spinal canal and avoids risk of thecal scarring. Furthermore, material enters the disc diagonally, away from the spinal canal and retropulsion would be less damaging. Being remote from the descending nerve root and lateral recess, relief of stenosis in this anatomy depends on restoring disc height.

Percutaneous Posterior Minimal Intervention Fenestration

Again using X-ray control a direct posterior approach is employed via a 2-cm incision. Purpose designed instrumentation allows soft tissue retraction by a

---

Hastings Orthopaedic Centre, Royal East Sussex Hospital, Hastings, East Sussex TN 34 1 ER, U.K.

The Artificial Disc
Ed. by M. Brock, H.M. Mayer and K. Weigel
© Springer-Verlag Berlin Heidelberg 1991

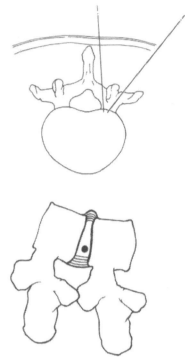

Fig. 1. Two minimal intervention approaches are described in the text, postero-lateral and postero-medial

Fig. 2. Bone graft dowels and piecemeal infill have been introduced percutaneously to achieve interbody fusion but the graft tends to crumble and fails to maintain re-establishment of disc height

lever applied over the facet joint, and a fibre optic suction root retractor provides a dry and illuminated interlamina access to the disc. Coaxial ascending access tubes, as in the blind access, are installed into the disc, up to a diameter of 1.4 cm. Therefore, a larger access portal is obtained, coupled with direct access to the nerve root in the lateral recess, but with the risk of possible scarring from manipulation of the theca. Also retropulsion of any intercorporal material would result in serious compromise of the spinal canal.

We undertook 15 percutaneous fusion procedures by the 45° postero-lateral approach using homograft piecemeal and bilateral dowel grafts (Fig. 2). Follow-up for 1 to 4 years indicated a good clinical result in only eight, definite radiological arthrodesis in only six, and loss of original post-operative disc height in 14 out of 15. Restoration of the lateral recess by the postero-lateral approach requires re-establishment of disc height, and we have now abandoned this technique as inadequate. However, no significant complications arose as a result of the access. Two problems contribute to the unreliable nature of the technique: (1) limited mechanical strength of graft bone, and (2) failure to eliminate movement. The diameter of any dowel can only be up to a maximum of the inner diameter of the access tube, thus leaving the system slack when the tube is removed. Lack of posterior fixation ensures continued movement about the graft which is at the fulcrum of motion in the segment.

As an alternative to homograft bone, intradiscal implants have been undergoing evaluation.

Intradiscal Implant

Fixation

The following devices are used in conjunction with hydroxyapatite ceramic slurry and homograft.

1. 1-cm expansion bullet (Fig. 3). This device is designed for introduction using the posterolateral percutaneous access. An outer diameter of 1-cm permits introduction via the 10-mm tube, and the split design allows subsequent introduction through the tube of an expansion tablet, of which three sizes are available. Bilateral implants, supplemented by posterior stapling of the facet joint, can be achieved via the percutaneous approach and appear to produce rigid and secure fixation.

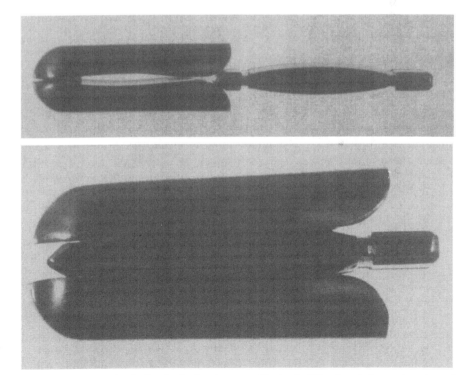

Fig. 3. An expansion bullet device has been used instead of the dowels for postero-lateral approach grafting

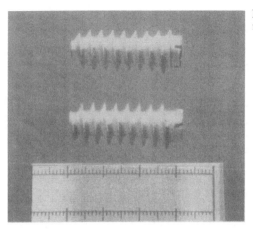

Fig. 4. HAC coated screw dowels may be used for postero-lateral fixation

2. Bilateral parallel 1.4-cm cancellous threaded dowels installed via the posterior MIF approach (Fig. 4). The diameter of the devices are sufficient to engage upper and lower plates, and laboratory studies suggest that secure fixation occurs without posterior fixation, but the danger of retropulsion is reduced by concurrent fixation of the facet joint at the same procedure using transfixing screws.

Disc Substitute

Whilst arthrodesis has the drawback of eliminating movement in one segment at the expense of the adjacent segment, greater potential hazards exist with a device which permits continuing movement, the most significant of which is formation of foreign body granulation material from wear products. For this reason these ideas must be seen as futuristic at he present time. The three methods described here await completion of animal studies before clinical application can be considered.

1. Shortened Intradiscal Bullet (Fig. 5). The bullet described and illustrated above has been shortened to half its original length and the flat ends of the expansion tablet removed. Shortened bullets are places in the nuclear area of the disc. Bilateral placement restores disc height and permits polycentric movement which minimises the natural disc. Laboratory tests suggest the arrangement is remarkably stable and bending stiffness and nuclear stability increase. The prototype material is titanium, but for clinical use ceramic will be required to reduce the risk of foreign body reaction.
2. Silastic Materials. Hollow dowels installed bilaterally into the nuclear zone, as in oblique placement of bone dowels described above, provide support and a more favourable annulus-nucleus loading ratio, but cyclic

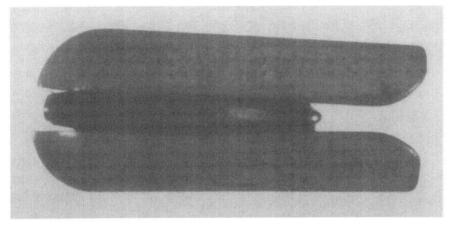

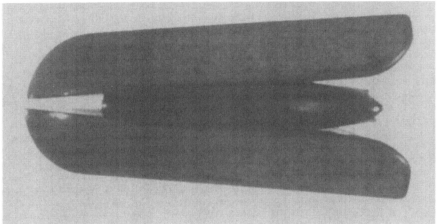

Fig. 5. A modified bullet can be used to permit continuing movement

loading in a test rig causes the dowels to migrate rather easily, perhaps due to lack of interference fit resulting from the dowel being of only the inside diameter of the tube. The curing of fluid silastic material in situ has the theoretical attraction that it would adopt the shape of the nucleus and thereby retain its position more effectively, although the physical conditions required for curing are either toxic at low temperature or requiring a temperature that is difficult to reproduce in biological tissues, and the resulting material would be faulty.

3. Hydrophylic Gels. These materials have been used in ophthalmology since being developed in 1964, both as contact lenses and prosthetic lens for cateract surgery. The dry gel bonds to between 30% and 70% of its own volume in water, expanding by a corresponding amount and changing to a pliable consistency. Original materials were of a resin base of hydroxyethylmethacrylate and the expanded structure has good

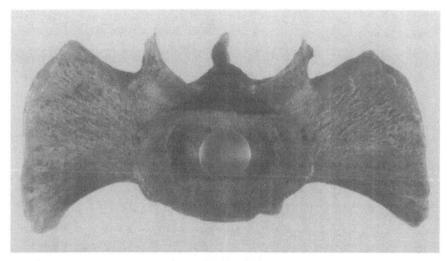

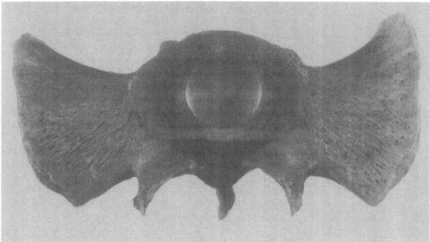

Fig. 6. Self-expanding hydrophilic jells are being investigated

compressive strength but very limited tensile strength and poor notch tear strength, and cannot sustain severe handling. Recent developments include hydrogels using styrene, nylon, methacrylate and acrylonitrile with more satisfactory mechanical properties. Materials of 50% water uptake can be either stiff or soft and elastic. Composite materials made for biomedical application use cross linked copolymers and are very stable. Systems can be fabricated using polyester fibre and polyamide cross linked copolymers with properties which approach that of nucleus pulposus. We are currently investigating these materials for wear and survivorship in vitro and the clear advantage of a material which expands to fill the gap left by disc excision means the implant has self-retaining qualities.

The natural history of most disc disorders trends towards eventual spontaneous resolution. Justification for surgical remedies at all remains questionable to a large proportion of both the lay public and our profession. Attempts to manufacture substitutes for biological materials and enthusiasm for technology must at all times be tempered by humility.

Lumbar Interbody Threaded Prostheses

C.D. RAY

Introduction

Two types of intradiscal prostheses are presented and discussed. They have been developed for two basic but opposite clinical-biomechanical reasons: (1) restoration or maintenance of discal height and mobility, viz., a prosthetic nucleus and (2) interbody fusion. Although at diametric ends of the mechanical spectrum, i.e., flexibile vs. rigid, both utilize a technique of threading (or tapping) holes bored or cut into the intradiscal or interbody space. The threaded external construction provides instant mechanical holding strength against expulsion of the prostheses and more than doubles the area of the interface contact, as compared with equivalent, smooth-surfaced devices. The flexible prosthetic nuclei require shallow threading of the vertebral end plates and no direct attachment to the bone, whereas the fusion devices must have deep penetration into bleeding spongiosa for ultimate ingrowth of vertebral bone.

The threaded outer shell of the flexible nuclei are woven of filaments, somewhat resembling segments of an aortic prosthesis; each has an internal, semipermeable membranous sac filled with hyaluronic acid and a thixotropic agent. Although inserted in a partly collapsed, relatively dehydrated, initial condition, the strongly hygroscopic hyaluronic acid within the capsular prosthesis swells rather rapidly, locks the matching threads of the device within the tapped recipient bed, and then continues to swell such that disc height and flexibility return. The formerly slack, partly degenerated anulus then tightens. The cyclic loading function, important to discal metabolism and caused by fluctuations in applied pressure (from body weight and muscle pull) balanced against swelling pressure of the nuclear gel, causes metabolites to leave and enter the disc. With primary functions thus restored, hopefully the anulus will heal. The viscosity altering thixotropic agent permits the contained fluid to translocate during bending, but take a set when immobile in order to imitate the normal rheology of the disc nucleus.

The rigid, threaded, titanium cage fusion devices have multiple perforations (60%−70%) around surfaces that penetrate well into the

---

Assoc. Director, Institute for Low Back Care, Minneapolis, MN 55407, USA

The Artificial Disc
Ed. by M. Brock, H.M. Mayer and K. Weigel
© Springer-Verlag Berlin Heidelberg 1991

54 C.D. RAY

threaded spongiosa. When packed with autologous, cancellous bone chips, a bony bridge grows across the cages and through the chips to unite the opposing vertebral bodies [35].

Anatomy and Biomechanics of the Normal Intervertebral Disc

Intervertebral discs, mechanical cushions of the axial skeleton, are unique structures comprising two principal types of tissue; an outer, multilayered ligamentous band; the anulus, built rather like a laminated automobile tire; and an inner, softer, partially movable, relatively amorphous, fibrocartilaginous nucleus. Each lumbar disc normally measures about 10–15 mm in height at rest but diminishes in height by 10%–25% on prolonged weight-bearing. The circumferential margin of the anular band is about 15 mm thick [19]. The contact surface area and size of the vertebral bodies vary linearly with the load carried; thus the average lowest lumbar dics have an area of about 20–28 cm2, becoming smaller with each higher disc [9]. The average size at the lumbosacral junction is about 3.5 × 5.5 cm. The fibers of the outer anulus, principally of type I collagen, are laid down in relatively discrete multiple layers; the fibers attach to the vertebral bodies at an angle of about 30°–40° in both directions, that is, right- and left-handed [37]. This design resists torsion, as half of these angulated fibers will tighten with vertebral rotation in either direction.

The discs comprise about 20% of the total length of the axial spine. The controlled motions between vertebral segments of the skeleton are determined and limited by flexibility of the discs, interverterbral ligaments, and by the facet joints. Although flexion-extension reaches about 12° per lumbar segment, lateral bending is about 5° and rotation is limited to about 1.5° [20, 32]. Greater freedom of rotation is potentially more destructive to the segmental structures and especially to emerging nerves [32, 43, 46].

As the vertebral column is bent and the end plates become out of parallel, compression or tension occurs on opposite sides of the anulus. This wedging motion is aided by a limited translocation of the semifluid internal nucleus away from the narrowed side [19, 45]. This translocation effects a shift in the center of motion between the vertebrae. The complex intervertebral motions demand both nuclear fluidity and anular flexibility and are important to anular integrity, as wedge bending is needed to reduce fiber stretch on the tension side [46].

The contained nucleus, acting rather like the fluid center of a golf ball, is strongly hygroscopic due to the mucopolysaccharide content. By imbibing water, this vaguely encapsulated, semifluid gel serves to keep the anulus tight (as does the air inside a tire); the gel also exhibits pressure-related swelling, viz., the nuclear fluid volume, which is reduced with gravity and muscular pull

[18]. Therefore, the discal height is determined by the total water content, which is at balance between applied pressure (body weight) and hygroscopic swelling pressure [3, 30, 35, 41]. The inner anulus and discal nucleus are the largest avascular, non-innervated structures of the body. Through cyclic loading, caused by fluctuations in applied force, fluid is exchanged (or pumped) between the internal disc and the vascularized vertebral end plates [37]. This hydraulic mechanism provides nutrition of and waste-product removal from the inner disc. Interestingly, this exchange occurs not across intact cartilagenous portions of the end plate, but through small perforations where segments of the nucleus and inner anulus penetrate [37]. Further, solutes of larger molecular species, e.g., albumin, globulins, glycogen, and proteins, do not cross the barrier [3, 16, 40]. Instead, the principal exchange is of water, ions, gases, some amino acids, and simple metabolites.

Normal lumbar intranuclear pressure under resting conditions has been measured at about 0.5 MPa (around 5 atmopheres or 75 psi); the pressure is more than tripled by exertion (especially when the spine is hyperextended) [15, 16, 41]. Resting pressure is perhaps 50% higher still in discs having degeneration and dehydration [1].

All body tissues show viscoelastic behavior, alterable by aging, disease, or disorder. Whenever the discal nucleus is degenerated, herniated, or removed by surgery, the disc space will narrow and lose part of its mobility [32, 42]. Resultant anular degeneration may predispose it to tearing of the fibers; an inflammatory condition may arise, resulting in motion pain of the anulus, i.e., discogenic pain [42, 46]. The complex sequence generally follows a pattern: As the nucleus loses its water-binding ability (similar to letting the air out of a tire), the height decreases and the anulus buckles; laminated plies begin to separate (delaminate) and radial tears may occur [1, 46]. Since the nucleus contains unique peptides, sealed since fetal life from the remainder of the body's circulating milieu, these tears permit contact between circulating immune globulins and the unique nuclear material [27]. It has been shown that autoimmune responses may result, producing both inflammation and further degeneration of the nucleus and inner anulus [29, 30].

Pertinent Biochemistry of the Disc

Mechanics of the disc largely depend on the organization of the extracellular matrix and the interaction between collagen, proteoglycans, and water. Proteoglycans have considerable influence on disc properties and functions. These large molecules have a protein core and abundant, attached chains of chondroitin and keratin sulphate [3]. Multimolecular aggregates are formed, together with hyaluronic acid, and further stabilized with a linking protein that helps to prevent dissociation of the aggregate [3, 18]. In several aspects, all articular hyaline cartilage has similar construction, but there are wide variations in the discal aggregates [3]. Further, aging changes occur earlier and more dramatically in discs than in other cartilages [3, 15, 18, 26]. Proteoglycans are constantly turned over by chondrocytes in the matrix [3, 27]. Thus, these cells are important to discal normalcy. There is a complex, closed feedback system for synthesis of discal proteoglycans; in short, the hydration of the disc (especially the nucleus) is dependent on proteoglycan content (among other things), and the degree of hydration influences chondrocytic synthesis of proteoglycans. It therefore appears essential that the hydration dependent discal height be at balance for normal intradiscal metabolism to proceed [27]. As hydration of the nucleus changes with cyclic loading, the concentration of solutes and metabolites will change. Therefore, all things considered, it is cyclic hydration of the disc space which holds a principal key to disc behavior and health.

Innervation of the Disc: Discogenic Pain and Anular Healing

The anulus is innervated only by A-delta and C fibers, which transmit pain and temperature sense. A weak sense of pressure is also transmitted. These sensations pass to the spinal cord by small somatic nerves that originate along the outside of the anulus, penetrating for a short distance (6–8 mm) inwardly across the fiber layers [4]. Abnormal shearing motion between these layers, due to loss of bonding between them, may stretch and irritate and free nerve endings. Certain changes in ionic concentration, caused by tissue injury or alteration in nerve cell permeability, may be sensed as pain. Mooney has shown that where the end plates have lost permeability due to degenerative changes, there may be an accumulation of acid metabolites within the nucleus; on traversing the anulus via tears these may serve as a pain stimulus [27]. I have found that by neutralizing these acid metabolites by injection of a small volume of NaOH at pH 8–10, most of the pain be temporarily eliminated. Thus, discal degeneration may permit chemical irritants to be pumped outward to excite or "inflame" anular nerves. Whatever the mechanism, the extreme sensitivity of the disc to movement may require either a reduction of the inflammation, an inhibition of the nerve excitability, or a mechanical limitation of the motion fusion in order to achieve clinical relief.

Like all other ligaments of the body, the anulus is capable of healing; however, mechanical and biochemical conditions must be appropriate [14]. For the motion sensitive, painfully disabling disc, even though the actual mechanical instability is minimal, the therapeutic choices are frequently limited; bony fusion may be the only present means to stop this micromotion-induced pain. It is the goal of the prosthetic nucleus to permit healing and thus restore anular function, hopefully preventing the need for a bony fusion. On the other hand, if the degeneration is too advanced, then a fusion, perhaps by means of the device presented below, may present a good clinical solution to segmental motion pain [34, 35].

Design and Function of the Prosthetc Lumbar Disc Nucleus

Prostheses have been used successfully in many joints to relieve painful, degenerative conditions. However, at present, no prosthetic disc is currently available for the combined purposes of maintaining or restoring: (a) disc height, (b) normal mechanical function, (c) cyclic swelling and, (d)

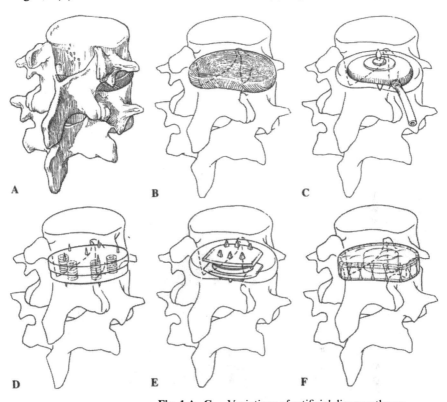

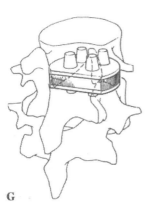

Fig. 1 A–G. Variations of artificial disc prostheses.
A Right posterolateral view of normal lumbar segments L4 and L5, for reference. **B** View as in A but with transparent bone. Normal L4–L5 interverbebral disc in position.
C Flexible, water-filled bladder attached by spikes to the bony end plates, (After [11]). **D** Overlapping metal plates with anchoring spikes. Note the internal springs. (After [31]). **E** Metal plates with end plate spikes. A high-density plastic sphere between the plates is a hinge about which the plates move. (After [6]). **F** Multilayered, fiber-reinforced, elastomeric wafer having 50%–80% the size of a normal disc. Tilted fibers imitate orientation of the natural anulus. Central elastomeric mass is highly compliant, with a progressive firmness distally. Bony attachment is somewhat unclear; losse fibers on outer surfaces are proposed mode. (After Stubstad, [22, 39]). **G** Porous metal plates and spikes separated by an elastomeric cushion. (After [38])

mechanical and biochemical circumstances amenable to anular healing (Fig. 1). The present prosthetic nucleus will attempt to achieve these goals [33, 35]. Clearly, prosthetic joints must become attached to bone to prevent displacement during motion. Disc prostheses to date require direct attachment to vertebral body bone by means of nailing, ingrowth into a porous metal or into polymeric fibers, or both [11, 12, 22, 35, 38]. The prosthetic device given here, lying within the nuclear cavity, requires only an indirect bony attachment. This is accomplished by the cutting of light threads in the end plates which match with the "threads" woven in the outer wall of the prostheses (Fig. 2). Shaped like small sausages, 12 mm diameter × 25 mm length, with a pitch of 10 threads per inch (2.5 mm thread distance), each threaded shell is a double-woven spiral of high tensile strength, flexible polymeric fibers, and tissue ingrowth-promoting filaments of polyglycolic acid (similar to absorbable suture material) [33, 35]. The mixed inert and active fibers become invaded by fibrous tissue of the lateral anulus as well as that of

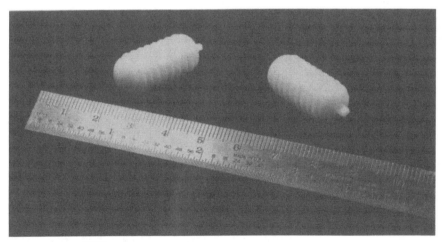

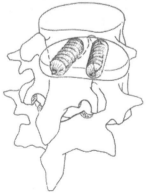

Fig. 2. A Woven, threaded, cylindrical, capsule prosthetic nucleus. (Courtesy CeDaR Surgical Inc. Minnetonka, MN 55345, USA). B Prosthetic nuclei in position, posterior insertion. (After [33, 35])

Lumbar Interbody Threaded Prostheses

the end plates. This invasion should preserve permanent flexibility of the implants without dependence on a rubbery elastomeric component. Such elastomeric polymers generally have a limited structural life in the hostile environment of the body.

The woven capsular structure of the prosthetic nucleus can withstand considerable applied pressure. The flexible, semipermeable, membranous sac inside each capsule contains a viscous, hygroscopic semifluid. With a thixotropic additive, the gel has freedom of movement with bending but resists movement during slow, postural changes, thereby promoting postural stability. Thus, the primary components together exhibit both cyclic loading and viscoelastic fluid translocation within the capsular prosthesis. All of the materials used in the prostheses are currently approved and are being used for human implantation; the combination of elements is quite unique, however.

Threaded Cages for Interbody Fusions

Intervertebral body (interbody) fusions result from the securing of graft material within the motion center of the vertebral segment. Thus, considerable biomechanical advantage occurs, as compared with posterior or intertransverse process fusions. The interbody fusion becomes both the central weight-bearing structure and a lock against segmental motion. On the other hand, it is technically simpler and safer to place grafts external to the disc. Principal among interbody fusion problems are: [1] Neurological deficit from nerve traction injury, due to pulling the roots or dura aside or compressing the ganglion during recipient bed preparation or while making room for insertion of the graft; [2] The need for considerable experience and skill in precise cutting of both the recipient site and graft (to prevent collapse or extrusion of the graft). In addition, virtual filling (about 75%) of the nucleus cavity with graft material is needed. Further, the use of bone itself brings additional technical problems, since although autologous, cancellous bone still remains the "gold standard" graft material, this relatively soft bone is often of insufficient strength to support the intervertebral space until fusion takes place. It is the attached cortical portion of these grafts that provide the vertical strength against collapse. Allograft bone, although considerably more plentiful, presents further burdens. Frozen-dried cadaver bone grafts are stronger than fresh grafts, albeit sometimes they are osteopenic and brittle; more importantly they may fail to incorporate into a fusion. Fresh frozen human bone may contain HIV or other transmissible viruses [21]. Whatever the graft material, it must in all cases have necessary strength and form to resist collapse or expulsion. Lastly, the patients' anatomy must be appropriate to the above demands, e.g., certain nerve roots cannot be fully retracted. The learning curve for these details may be quite long.

A number of substitute or prosthetic material have been developed to circumvent the need for autologous bone. They include animal bone,

60 C.D. RAY

hydroxyapatite formulations, sea coral, porous ceramics, composites, and cancellous metal [5, 10, 27, 44]. Results to date indicate that the preferred material is yet to be found; other than autologous bone.

The prevention of graft expulsion, especially during flexion-extension of the lumbar spine, has received considerable attention. For example, tapered, tricortical pelvic bone grafts and matching recipient beds, used in posterior lumbar interbody fusions (PLIF), require that the taper must be largest deep inside the intervertebral space. The depth of cut (purchase) into each vertebra must provide good bivertebral bony exposure. Several instrument systems are available to facilitate these tedious cutting processes [7, 8, 23, 25, 28, 47]. Nevertheless, dislodgement of the grafts occurs in 2%–10% of patients [8, 23, 25, 28]. As the rectangular beds are cut and grafts placed, retraction of the superior, lateral corners of the laminotomies by cutters, chisels, and grafts present a considerable hazard to nerves [28, 36]. Round holes are easier to cut, but strong, matching bone grafts are not easily harvested. Threading the bone grafts and beds as a means to prevent expulsion has been described for cervical fusions [43].

Although several methods have been developed to assure the success of lumbar interbody fusions, the failure rates vary widely, from 5% to 70%; the complication rate may also be rather high, especially among newcomer surgeons [23, 25, 28]. Further, some grafts may show invasion by remnant, intradiscal soft tissue from the lateral aspect of the graft; until now this route could not be blocked [14].

The New Interbody Concept

Cylindrical, multiple perforated metal cylinders were developed for long bone fusions by Longfellow [24]. Later, interbody fusion "baskets" were developed by the orthopaedist George Bagby to be used in the cervical spine of horses afflicted with subluxation, cord compression, and paresis, called the "wobbler" syndrome [2, 10]. Bagby's baskets are made from stainless steel tubes into which many holes are unformly drilled (up to about 30% of the outer wall surface). These multiperforate steel cylinders are driven tightly into a hole bored into the spongiosae of opposing vertebrae; they are then filled with autologous bone chips. The horses' cervical discs are quite thin (2–4 mm). As the bone grows through the baskets and across to the other vertebra, a strong union develops in about 88% of the animals [10]. The Bagby concept has considerable merit in that the cylinder (only one is placed, from an anterior approach) maintains strength against collapse as the fusion develops (locking the basket into the fusion.) Further, the volume of unformed autologous bone is small (about 10 ml). Since the baskets are round, the recipient hole is easily drilled. Even though a basket is driven tightly into an undersized hole, about 7% dislodge [10]. Further, some of the recipient vertebrae fracture or show pressure necrosis with fibrous halo formation around the implant.

Threaded Cages and Instruments

The new fusion device presented here is a thin walled, threaded tubular shell of titanium (Fig. 3A). The fusion "cage" may then be simply screwed into a previously drilled and tapped (threaded) bivertebral hole. A pair of such cages is implanted by a modified, simplified PLIF technique [36]. Once seated, 5 ml of soft, autologous, cancellous bone is packed inside each seated cage and a plastic retaining cap applied. The fusion develops by ingrowth from both opposing spongiosae. The threads which are cut along the outer walls of the cages break through the apices of internal arches, creating large

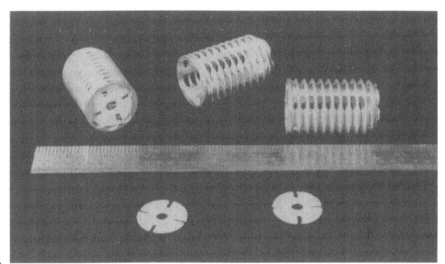

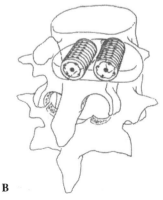

Fig. 3. **A** Threaded fusion cages with end caps. Note high porosity and thinness of threaded walls. (Courtesy CeDaR Surgical Inc. Minnetonka, MN 55345, USA). **B** Threaded cages in position, posterior insertion. (After [36])

(1.5 × 4.0 mm) perforations; the cage shell is about 70% perforated on the superior and inferior sides, i.e., only along the surfaces that penetrate into the spongiosae. The sides presenting to the intradiscal space are blocked to prevent fibrous tissue from growing into the graft. The unusual shape also contributes to the high strength of the device. The measured deformation strength of an individual titanium cage, in a simulated clinical circumstance, was over 425 kg, greater than four to five times the strength of healthy human vertebrae. Cages cyclically loaded to 200 kg for over million cycles have not shown mechanical failure. The round cylinder makes the cutting drilling, and threading of the recipient hole quite gentle and simple; the threaded construction prohibits expulsion. A special C-shaped retractor, placed into a semicircular laminotomy, holds the neural tissues aside and internally guides the drilling and threading elements. This split tubular retractor presents a smooth, superior, lateral surface to the nerve and is far less likely to cause neural compression. The cages and recipient bone are not tapered or hammered. A pair of cages placed bilaterally (Fig. 3B) limits all motions, except axial of the segment, which is held by body weight and elastic recoil of tissues (stretched before the space is drilled).

The autologous, cancellous particulate graft bone is taken from a nearby posterior iliac spine. Although the fusion is created later by the traversing growth of bone, there is immediate stabilization of the disc space. The large, oval perforations should prohibit stress shielding of the contained bone; that is, the bone should simply penetrate the oval holes more deeply as settling and remodeling occur. The procedure has been safe, sure and rapid and generally requires under 3 h to perform a single, bilateral level.

Surgical Techniques

The surgical approaches and methods of insertion of both threaded devices are quite similar, differing primarily in the overlying tissue (ligament and bone) removed, appropriate to the size of the device. Cages vary in size (14, 16, 18 mm maximum outside diameter); an additional 1.5 mm diameter, in the semicircular laminotomy, is needed to accommodate the outside diameter of the C retractor. Since the space must remain under static tension, the disc space is spread widely; this requires the removal of the interpinous and flavum ligaments. Thus, elastic recoil of the anulus, pull of muscles, and gravity hold the cages in position until fused.

On the other hand, since the threaded nucleus halves are self-inflating and create their own counterforce, the removal of posterior ligaments is not needed. A standard laminotomy for discectomy suffices. In their initial, dehydrated state, the prosthetic nuclei are 20 mm long, 8 and 10 mm in outside diameter; the recipient beds are no larger. When fully inflated by tissue water, they will rise 2–4 mm (intradiscal height), in a balance between swelling and applied pressures. The dorsal discal surface should be exposed

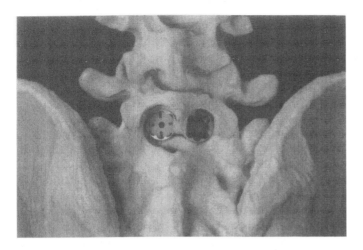

Fig. 4. Human spine model showing threaded fusion cages in position; posterior cap applied and removed. Note internal arcuate structure of cages, with blockage of lateral walls adjacent to disc space. Also note proximity of cages to overlying each other

bilaterally and a core of disc removed using a pilot drill. On inspecting inside the hole, both end plates should be equally but lightly penetrated by an appropriate core drill even if one finds a significant Schmorl "dome" in the discal center. A tap of correct size lightly threads the end plates along the majority of their opposing surfaces. A dehydrated prosthesis of suitable diameter is placed inside the tapped hole and irrigated until it begins to expand. The external nipple permits maneuvering of the capsule to match the cut threads as well as testing the pullout strength, as shown in Fig. 2B. The patient is braced lightly and a lateral plain film made at closure and daily for 3 days. If all goes well, patients should be able to resume progressive activities after weeks.

For the cage fusions, the technique is clearly more complex. The interspinous and flavum ligaments are removed, the laminas are distracted, and a limited laminotomy is made. Again, a pilot drill is drilled into the disc space, seeking the discal midline. A pilot rod then replaces the drill. A circular lamina cutter, passed over the pilot rod, laterally cuts the spinous process and scores the lamina. A bone punch or turbine is used to cut away the scored lamina, making a semicircular laminotomy, facetectomy, and pediclotomy. With the dura and nerve carefully maneuvered aside, the C retractor is placed through the semicircular hemilaminotomy and lodged into the dorsum of the vertebral bodies. Drilling and threading of the vertebrae and the insertion of the cage 48 are then completed. All tools are marked for depth control. The second side is similarly done. Chips of cancellous bone, taken from a nearby iliac spine, are tightly packed into the cages and small plastic caps are applied to retain the bone chips (Fig. 4). Flexion is limited by tying a 5 mm Mersilene polyester tape, figure eight style, around the bases of the two dorsal processes. The wound is closed and drained. Blood loss has been under 250 ml in most patients.

Clinical Experience

Ten patients have been implanted with threaded fusion cages; five were at the L5-S1 level alone, three at L4-5 alone (one patient had spontaneous collapse and rigidity at L5-S1); one was for a floating fusion at the L3-4 level alone, and one required a two level procedure (L4-5 and L5-S1). Patients (8 male, 2 female) had an average age of 38 years and had been screened using both CT and facet joint screening injections and provocative discography (using saline and subsequent contrast media) into the involved segments. The latter test injections confirmed the diagnosis of discogenic pain. Three of our patients had prior discectomies at one of the cage implant segments. One patient had a failed posterolateral fusion procedure. The postoperative follow-up period to date ranges from 9 to 17 months. One patient had lateral stenosis, resulting in leg pain greater than back pain. This patient underwent

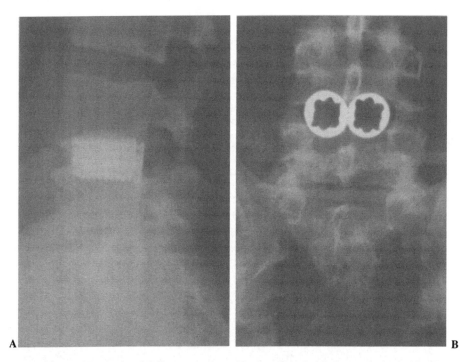

Fig. 5 A,B. **A** Lateral and **B** Ferguson views showing threaded fusion cages in position for "floating" fusion at L4-L5 level. Darker "halo" around the cages is due to circular cutting of posterior laminae. (Compare with Fig. 4)

Lumbar Interbody Threaded Prostheses 65

a bilateral decompression at the collapsed, rigid level (L5–S1), and cages were implanted at the discogenic pain level (L4–5). This 33 year old man has reported greater than 90% relief of both back and leg symptoms since the first postoperative week. Figure 5 shows AP and lateral postimplant films of this patient. To dale all 10 cases have shown fusion of the cage-implanted segments. As yet, no patient has received the prosthetic nuclei. Current work has been devoted to invitro mechanical and physicochemical testing.

Clinical courses of all but one fusion cage patients to date have been remarkable. They have reported early, good to excellent relief of their original low back pain. The exceptional patient had four prior surgeries and has not returned to work in 7 years; his cages appear stable and unchanged after 4 months; flexion-extension films show no motion in the fused segment. This man treated in a pain rehabilitation clinic. Three patients have had postoperative CT scans; two, an MRI. These imaging studies showed considerable metal artifacts, although less than in patients with pedicle screw and plate implants. The MRI scans are remarkably free of artifact, however. All patients agreed to refrain from any use of tobacco for several weeks before and 6 months after surgery.

Discussion

The two new implantable devices and surgical methods use threading of their structures to prevent dislodgement or expulsion. The pair of woven, filled, hygroscopic, capsular nucleus prostheses are designed to restore discal height and flexibility, hopefully permitting the anulus to heal. The highly perforated metal cages, screwed between drilled and tapped adjacent vertebral bodies and then packed with cancellous bone, were developed for interbody fusions. The fusion technique has shown early clinical promise, although no prosthetic disc has yet been implanted. Longer follow-up will determine the ultimate fate of the fusions. Non-metal cages (ceramic or plastic composite construction) are under development for radiographic and magnetic invisibility. Cages of larger diameter for anterior interbody use are now being readied.

Acknowledgements. The prostheses and surgical instruments (patents pending) were developed together with CeDaR Surgical, Inc., Minnetonka, MN, 55343, USA. The author thanks his colleagues at the Institute for Low Back Care, especially his associate, Dr. Richard Salib, and his physician's assistant, Matthew Garner, for help, encouragement, and suggestions. Appreciation is also extended to Gene Dickhudt for his expertise in instrument development and Lavern Hennum for the expert machining of cages. The cages and associated surgical instruments are now made by Surgical Dynamics, Inc., Alameda, CA, USA. CeDaR Development Corp. makes the prosthetic nuclei.

References

1. Adams MA, Hutton WC (1985) Gradual disc prolapse. Spine 10: 524–531
2. Bagby GW (1987) Stainless steel implants for intervertebral body fusions. North Am Spine Soc, Proc Ann Meet, Paper #34, pp 89–90, June 27
3. Bayliss, MT, Johnstone B, O'Brien JP (1988) Proteoglycan synthesis in the human intervertebral disc: Variation with age, region and pathology. Spine 13: 972–981
4. Bogduk N, Tynan W, Wilson AS (1981) The nerve supply to the human lumbar intervertebral discs. J Anat 132: 39–56
5. Brantigan JW (1988) Surgical prosthetic implant facilitating vertebral interbody fusion and method. US Patent Office, Patent No. 4,743,256, May 10
6. Buettner-Janz K, Schellnack K, Zippel H (1987) Eine alternative Behandlungsstrategie beim lumbalen Bandscheibenschaden mit der Bandscheibenendoprothese Modulartyp SB Charite. Z Orthop 125: 1–6
7. Cloward RB (1953) The treatment of ruptured lumbar intervertebral discs by vertebral body fusion. J Neurosurg 10: 154–166
8. Collis JS (1985) Total disc replacement: a modified posterior lumbar interbody fusion. Clin Orthop 193: 64–71
9. Columbini D, Occhipinti E, Grieco A, Faccini M (1989) Estimation of lumbar disc areas by means of anthropometric parameters. Spine 14: 51–55
10. DeBowes RN, Grant BD, Bagby GW Gallina AM, Sande RD, Ratzlaff MH (1984) Cervical vertebral interbody fusion in the horse: a comparitive study of bovine xenografts and autologous supported by stainless steel baskets. Am J Vet Res 45: 191–199
11. Froning EC (1975) Intervertebral disc prosthesis and instruments for locating same. US Patent Office, Patent No. 3,875,595, Apr 8
12. Goel VK, Nishiyama K, Weinstein JN, Liu YK (1986) Mechanical properties of lumbar spinal motion segments as affected by partial disc removal. Spine 11: 1008–1012
13. Goel VK, Kim YE, Lim T-H, Weinstein JN (1989) An analytical investigation of the mechanics of spinal instrumentation. Spine 14
14. Goodship AE, Wilcox SA, Shah JS (1985) The development of tissue around various prosthetic implants used as replacements for ligaments and tendons. Clin Orthop 196: 61–68
15. Holm S, Maroudas A, Urban JPG, Selstam G, Nachemson A (1981) Nutrition of the intervertebral disc: solute transport and metabolism. Connect Tissue Res 8: 101–119
16. Keller TS, Hansson TH, Holm SH, Pope MM, Spengler DM (1989) In vivo creep behavior of the normal and degenerated porcine intervertebral disk: a preliminary report. J Spinal Disord 1: 267–278
17. Kostuik, JP (1989) Artificial disc. (Camp Inc., Jackson MI), Back Issues 2(2): 1–2
18. Kraemer J, Kolditz D, Gowin R (1985) Water and electrolyte content of human intervertebral discs under variable load. Spine 10: 69–71
19. Krag MH, Seroussi RE, Wilder DG, Pope MH (1987) Internal displacement from in vitro loading of human thoracic and lumbar spinal motion segments: experimental results and theoretical predictions. Spine 10: 1001–1007
20. Kunz JD (1982) Intervertebral disc prosthesis. US Patent Office, Patent No. 4,349,921, Sep 21
21. Leads from the MMWR (1988) Transmission of HIV through bone transplantation case report and Public Health recommendations. JAMA 260: 2487–2489
22. Lee CK, Langrana NA, Alexander H, Clemow, AJ, Chen EH, Parsons JR, Yang SW (1989) Fiber-reinforced functional disc prosthesis. (abstr) Orthop Res Soc, Proc Ann Meet, Las Vegas, NV
23. Lin PM et al (1983) Posterior lumbar interbody fusion. Clin Orthop 180: 154–165
24. Longfellow EE (1951) Surgical appliance and method for fixation of bone fragments. US Patent Office, Patent No. 2,537,070, Jan 9

Lumbar Interbody Threaded Prostheses

25. Ma GW (1985) Posterior lumbar interbody fusion with specialized instruments. Clin Orthop 193: 57–74
26. Miller JAA, Schmatz C, Schultz AB (1988) Lumbar disc degeneration: Correlation with age, sex and spine level in 600 autopsy specimens. Spine 13: 173–178
27. Mooney V (1989) A perspective on the future of low back research. In: Guyer RD (ed), Spine: State of the Art Reviews. Philadelphia, Hanley & Belfus, 3: 173–183
28. Mosdal C (1985) Cervical osteochondrosis and disc herniation. Eighteen years use of interbody fusion by Cloward's technique in 755 cases. Acta Neurochirurgica 70: 207–225
29. Naylor A, Happey F, Turner RL, Shendall RD, West DC, Richardson C (1975) Enzymatic and immunological activity in the intervertebral disc. Orthop Clin No Amer 6: 51–58
30. Naylor A (1976) Intervertebral disc prolapse and degeneration: The biochemical and biophysical approach. Spine 1: 108–114
31. Patil AA (1982) Artificial intervertebral disc. US Patent Office, Patent No. 4,309,777, Jan 12
32. Pearcy MJ, Tibrewal SB (1984) Axial rotation and lateral bending in the normal lumbar spine measured by three-dimensional radiography. Spine 9: 582–587
33. Ray CD, Corbin T (1988) Prosthetic disc and method of implanting. US Patent Office, Patent No. 4,772,287 (additional US and foreign patents pending), Sep 20
34. Ray CD (1988) Transfacet decompression and dowel fixation: A new technique for lumbar lateral spinal stenosis. Acta Neurochirurgica (Suppl) 43: 48–54
35. Ray CD (1988) Artificial disc. (abstr) p 67, Challenge of The Lumbar Spine, Proc Ann Meet, San Antonio, TX
36. Ray CD (1989) Threaded fusion cage: new technique for lumbar interbody fusions. (abstract, poster display) North Am Spine Soc, Ann Meet, Quebec City, June 29
37. Roberts S, Menage J, Urban JPG (1989) Biochemical and structural properties of the cartilage end–plate and its relation to the intervertebral disc. Spine 14: 166–174
38. Steffe A (1988) Artificial disc. (abstr) p 66, Challenge of The Lumbar Spine, Proc Ann Meet, San Antonio, TX
39. Stubstad JA, Urbaniak JR, Kahn P (1975) Prosthesis for spinal repair. US Patent Office, Patent No. 3,867,728, Feb 25
40. Tanz SS (1953) Motion of the lumbar spine: A roentgenologic study. Am J Roentg 69: 399–412
41. Urban JPG, McMullin JF (1988) Swelling pressure of the lumbar intervertebral discs: Influence of age, spinal level, composition and degeneration. Spine 13: 179–187
42. Vanharanta H, Sachs BL, Spivey M, Hochschuler SH, Guyer RD, Rashbaum RF, Ohnmeiss DD, Mooney V (1988) A comparison of CT/discography, pain response and radiographic disc height. Spine 13:321–324
43. Vich JMO (1985) Anterior cervical interbody fusion with threaded cylindrical bone. J Neurosurg 63: 750–753
44. Waisbrod H (1988) Treatment of metastatic disease of the spine with anterior resection and stabilization by means of a new cancellous metal construct. Arch Orth Trauma Surg 107: 222–225
45. White AA, Panjabi MM (1978) The basic kinematics of the human spine. Spine 3: 12–20
46. Wilder DG, Pope MH, Frymoyer JW (1988) The biomechanics of disc herniation and the effect of overload and instability. J Spinal Disord 1: 16: 32
47. Wiltberger BR (1964) Intervertebral body fusion by the use of posterior bone dowels. Clinical Orthopedics 35: 69–79

"Charité Modular":
Conception, Experience and Results

H. ZIPPEL

The late postoperative results of conventional disc surgery are frequently moderate or poor due to the consequent narrowing of the intervertebral space and intervertebral foramen [8], secondary incongruities and osteoarthrotic changes of facet joints [13], and alteration of the kinetic center [12] with more or less painful instability of the movable spinal segment.

After fusion of the degenerated segment, solid stabilization is the best way to obtain restoration of the intervertebral space at this level; however fusion inceases overload and stress in neighboring segments with the danger of premature wear and progressive destruction [14, 15]. Restoration of the intervertebral disc by means of an endoprosthesis should prevent secondary changes adjacent levels, provided that the artificial disc has the same biomechanical and functional properties as the orginal disc. These are:

- distance protection of the intervertebral space
- realization and maintenance of normal motion of the movale segment
- shock damping or shock absorption under peak axial load.

The theory, of intervertebral disc replacement was first reported in 1956 by van Steenbrugghe [23]. Between 1964 and 1967, Fernström, in Sweden, implanted 267 steel ball endoprostheses in the cervical and lumbar spine 195 patients after disc removal by posterior approach. Harmon (1961) [8], Reitz and Joubert (1964) [18], and Mc Kenzie (1971) [16] were among those who, in the 1950s and 1960s implanted steel balls into the intervertebral spaces in a number of patients. Long-term results with this ball prosthesis were relatively unsuccessful, as the steel ball migrated into the adjacent vertebral body end plates under axial load. After 4−7 years only 12% of Fernström's ball prostheses had an unchanged intervertebral distance [7]. Moreover, the ball prosthesis leads to uncontrolled and unphysiological movement in the movable spine segment with secondary alterations of the facet joints.

Flexible silicone plastics for disc replacement have been tried but with little success [4, 5, 6, 9, 10, 11, 19, 20, 21, 22, 24]. This applies to all types of silicon rubber without material-specific limitations. They are also unsuitable

---

Klinik und Poliklinik für Orthopädie, Bereich Medizin (Charité), Humboldt-Universität, Schumannstr. 20−21, O-1040 Berlin, FRG

The Artificial Disc
Ed. by M. Brock, H.M. Mayer and K. Weigel
© Springer-Verlag Berlin Heidelberg 1991

for such important surgical aims as restoration of intervertebral distance and elimination of facet joints subluxation.

Our own disc endoprosthesis developed in 1982, consists of three parts:

– Two central concave molded metallic plates with spikes or teeth to be fixed without cement to the vertebral body end-plates. The metallic material used initially was stainless steel and later a cobalt-chromalloy (ISO 5832/IV)
– Interposed between both metallic plates is a biconvex lenticular slide core of high-density polyethylene (Chirulen, Hoechst AG, FRG) as interspace filling material.

The polyethylene core has a ring-like wall to limit motion and prevent luxation of the lens core under movement and load. In addition the lens core is produced in various heights. The metallic wire-ring, which surrounds the polyethylene core, serves only for X-ray identification.

The material combination is in conformity with a low-friction principle. Mode and limitation of mobility correspond approximately to the physiological movement in the lower lumbar spine. The shock-damping properties of the artificial disc are limited by properties of the polyethylene material, its aging, especially the "cold-flow".

Static and dynamic studies of the artificial disc were carried out using a servohydraulic test rig. In static testing we obsrved hysteresis (hysteresis loops) in the polyethylene slide core in response to up to 2.4 kN. Loads between 6 and 8 kN produced incipient irreversible deformation, and loads over 10.5 kN reduced the slide core height by about 10%. Dynamic behavior was tested with 5–10 cyles per second and a deflction about neutral position $\pm$ 10° over 2 × 10^7 cyles, which corresponds to an equivalent of 20 years of use. Under these conditions, slide cores deformed by about 10% within the first 2 "equivalent years". Cadaveric testing showed migration and fracture of vertebral body end plates or vertebral destruction, depending on the disc model of used, between 4 and 8 kN (SB I) and up to 10 kN (SB II) (3).

After observing implant-specific failures and complications during clinical use, we have changed and modified our implant design three times. The first model (SB I) had circular stainless steel plates with 11, and later five, spikes fied to the disc endoprosthesis vertebral bodies (Fig. 1). In the following model (SB II), the anchoring surface of the stainless steel parts was increased by means of lateral wings (Fig. 2). The present model (SB III), produced by W. Link, (Hamburg, FRG) has stable and anatomically designed metallic end plates of various sizes made of cobalt-chromeally (ISO 5832/IV) (Fig. 3).

We started surgical implantation in September 1984 and have now implanted more than 100 artificial discs in the lumbar spine.

The disc endoprosthesis is implanted using an anterior approach. We prefer a left extraperitoneal route. The anterior longitudinal spinal ligament

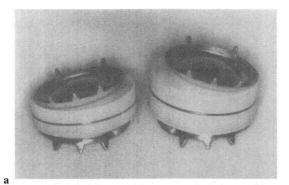

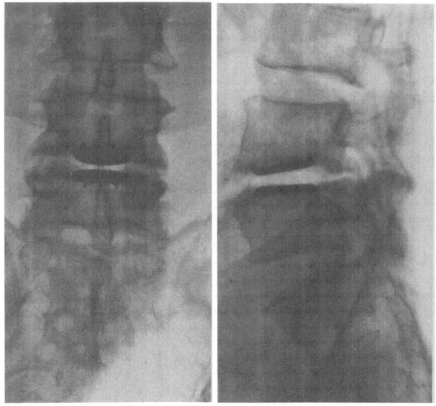

Fig. 1. a Artificial disc model SB I with polyethylene lens core in various sizes. **b** X-ray follow-up 3 years postoperatively in a 49-year-old male patient. Partial migration of the metallic part of the implant into the cranial end plate and slow ossification of the anulus fibrosus is shown

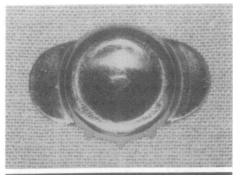
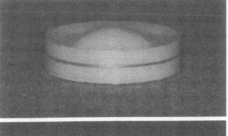
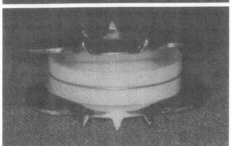

Fig. 2. **a** Artificial disc model SB II with enlarged metallic end plate (*top*) typical lens core (*center*), and complete disc (*bottom*). **b** Two years postoperatively in a 54-year-old man, complete ossification and fusion of the operated movable segment

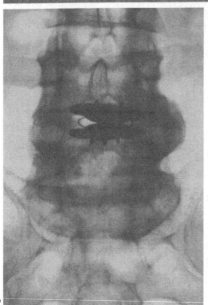
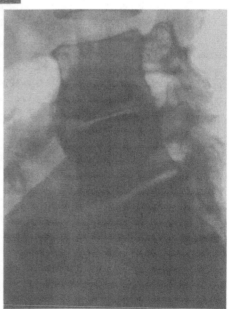

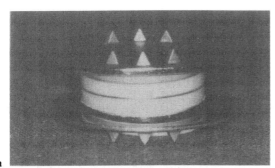

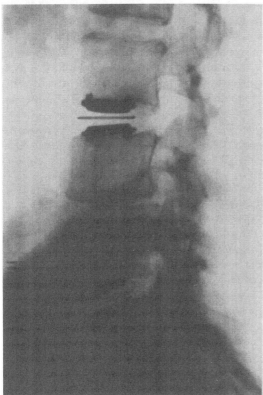

Fig. 3. a Model of the disc endoprosthesis (SB III) produced by W. Link (Hamburg, FRG). **b** Lateral X-ray follow-up of a 44-year-old male after replacement of L 3/4 and L 5/S 1, 1 year postoperative

is opened door-wing-like. Degenerative disc tissue is removed, a mild curettage of the vertebral body end plates is performed, and the intervertebral space is spread apart with a modified Scaglietti forceps. The size of the vertebral body end plates is measured with special instruments and the definitive position of the artificial disc prepared. Finally, the implant is inserted under and X-ray monitoring, in an anteroposterior and lateral approach. The forceps is removed, and the teeth of the artificial disc attach

74 H. ZIPPEL

themselves to the vertebral bodies. The anterior ligament is sutured and the wound is closed.

The operation requires an average of 50–60 min. The loss of blood is 200–300 ml. The duration of the procedure depends on the difficulties related to the surgical approach (large vessels!). The postoperative care is of short duration and simple. Patients stand 1 day after the operation and receive physiotherapy with special exercises to strengthen their back and stomach muscles. The hospital stay is approximately 16 days.

Main indications for artificial disc replacement are painful monosegmental or oligosegmental disc degenerations with or without instabilities after failure of conservative treatment or painful back syndromes after disc herniated operations, ("failed backs").

Contraindications are: osteoporosis, narrow spinal channel syndromes, severe spondylolisthesis, severe osteoarthrosis of facet joints, deficient ability and readiness to cooperate, psychic disorders, and latent spinal infections. A prerequisite for artificial disc implantation is high stability of the vertebral body end plates. For that reason, osteoporotic changes of the spine are absolute contra indications.

Important in the preoperative diagnosis is the detection of the cause of pain and segmental localization of the pain-producing segment. Our diagnostic assessment includes:

– Clinical and neurologicl examination
– X–ray examination in normal and bending positions
– Myelography (to exclude a free prolapse)
– Discography (not only to see the degenerative disc, but also, above all, for induction of memory pain – the best possible way to identify the pain-producing spinal segment)
– CT scan to estimate the condition of facet joints
– MRI

Materials and Results

Between 1984 and 1987, we implanted 76 artificial discs in 62 patients (23 men, 39 women). Average age of the patients was 43 years (min. 26 years, max. 59 years). Of these 23 patients had a failed operative therapy (37 nucleotomies); 39 patients had an unsuccessful conservative therapy before disc implantation. Segmental localization of disc replacement and artificial disc models used are shown in Tables 1 and 2.

We performed 48 monosegmental and 14 bisegmental disc replacements. In 6 patients we observed general post-operative complications (two disturbed wound healings, two urinary infections, and two deep-vein thromboses). Follow-up examination of all patients (between 15 months and 3 years postoperatively) showed a mean segmental mobility of artificial discs of 5°

"Charité Modular": Conception, Experience and Results

Table 1. Segmental localization of artificial disc replacement (n = 76)

Segment	n
L 2/3	1
L 3/4	4
L 4/5	41
L 5/S 1	30

Table 2. Implanted disc models (n = 76)

Model	n
SB I	14
SB II	44
SB III	18

Table 3. Intervertebral space before and after artificial disc replacement

	Normal	Decreased
Preoperative	13%	87%
Postoperative	84%	17%

(preoperative mobility: 9°) in sagittally bending X-rays. The intervertebral space was normalized or enlarged in the majority of patients (Table 3).

In 10 patients, there were migrations or dislocations of implants or vertebral body infractions; in 17 patients we observed stress or fatigue fractures of metallic parts of the artificial discs; and in four patients it was necessary to remove the implant and perform a secondary fusion. The results regarding pain, complaints, movement, and ability to work, taken from a subjective evaluation of the patients, were: very good, 54%; better, 29%; unchanged, 15%; and poor, 2%.

Finally, assessing the merits or demerits of endoprosthetic disc replacement, I can point out the principle advantages of using artificial discs in comparison to conventional nucleotomy or segmental fusion of the spine:

- maintenance of movable segments
- abolition of instability
- normalization of the intervertebral space
- enlargement of the intervertebral foramen.

Disadvantages are a indication and, up to now, a considerable number of implant failures with our model. Of course, since we have been using only the SB-III-model, we have not seen any fatigue fractures of metallic end plates, but we must continue to watch for migrations of metallic end plates into the vertebral bodies. This complication was also reported by Witting et al. (1989). It seems that both, implant fractures and implant migrations are caused by the quite different elasticity of the artificial disc, on the one hand and of the normal movable segment, on the other. Thus, further development of endoprosthetic design must start here. Another open question and a general problem in disc replacemet surgery is the importance of facet joints, as an essential part of the movable spinal segment, in recurrent pain after surgery.

76   H. ZIPPEL

We must probably pay greater attention in the future to the facet joints if we want a substantial improvement in long–term results of lumbar discre placement.

References

1. Büttner-Janz K, Schellnack K, Zippel H (1987) Eine alternative Behandlungsstrategie beim lumbalen Bandscheibenschaden mit der Bandscheibenendoprothese Modular-typ SB Charité. Z Orthop 125: 1–6
2. Büttner-Janz K, Schellnack K, Zippel H, Conrad P (1988) Erfahrungen und Ergebnisse mit der lumbalen Zwischenwirbel-Endoprothese SB Charité. Z Klin Med 43: 1785–1789
3. Büttner-Janz K, Schellnack K, Zippel H (1988) Biomechanics of the SB Charité lumbar intervertebral disc endoprosthesis. Intern Orthopaedics (SICOT) 13: 173–176
4. Edeland HG (1982) Suggestions for a total elasto–dynamic inter–vertebral disc prosthesis. Biomat Med Devices Artif Organs 9: 65–72
5. Edeland HG (1985) Some additional suggestions for an intervertebral disc prosthesis. J Biomed Eng 7: 57–62
6. Fassio B, Ginestie JF (1978) Prothèse discale en silicone. Etude experimental et premiéres observations cliniques. Nouv Presse Med 21: 207
7. Fernström U (1972) Der Bandscheibenersatz mit Erhaltung der Beweglichkeit. In: Junghanns H (Hrsg) Die Wirbelsäule in Forschung und Praxis, Bd 55 Hippokrates, S125–130, Stuttgart
8. Harmon PH (1961) Anterior extraperitoneal lumbar disc excision and vertebral body fusion. Clin Orthop 16: 169
9. Hirayama Y, Ojima S, Tkata H, Matsuzaki H (1988) Artificial intervertebral disc. FP O 317.972 A 1–23.11
10. Hoffmann–Daimler S (1974) Zur Frage des Bandscheibenersatzes. Z Orthop 112: 792–795
11. Horst M (1982) Mechanische Beanspruchung der Wirbelkörperdeckplatte. In: Junghanns H (Hrsg) Die Wirbelsäule in Forschung und Praxis Bd 95. Hippokrates, Stuttgart
12. Kapanji, JA (1985) Funktionelle Anatomie der Gelenke, Bd 3: Rumpf und Wirbelsäule. In: Otte P, Schlegel KF (Hrsg) Bücherei des Orthopäden, Bd 48. Enke, Stuttgart
13. Krämer J (1986) Bandscheibenbedingte Erkrankungen, 2 Aufl. Thieme, Stuttgart New York
14. Kreusche-Brinker R, Grober W, Mark P (1986) Die ventrale interkoporelle Spondylodese bei lumbaler Instabilität. Z Orthop 124: 619–627
15. Lee CK, Langrana NA (1984) Lumbosacral spinal fusion: a biomechanical study. Spine 9: 574–581
16. Mc Kenzie: Zit. in: Fernström U (1972) [7]
17. Nachemson A (1962) Some mechanical properties of the lumbar intervertebral discs. Bull Hosp Joint Dis 23: 130–143
18. Reitz H, Joubert MJ (1964) Intractable headache and cervico-brachialgia treated by complete replacement of cervical intervertebral discs with a metal prothesis. South Afr Med J 38: 881–884
19. Roy-Camille R, Saillant G, Lavaste F (1978) Etude expérimental d' un replacement discal lombaire. Rev Chir Orthop (Suppl 2) 64: 106–107
20. Schneider PG, Oyen R (1974) Bandscheibenersatz. Experimentelle Untersuchungen – Klinische Konsequenzen. Z Orthop 112: 791–792
21. Schneider PG, Oyen R (1974) Plastische Bandscheibenchirurgie. Bandscheibenersatz im lumbalen Bereich mit Silikonkautschuk. Theoretische und experimentelle Unter-suchungen. Z Orthop 112: 1078–1086

"Charité Modular": Conception, Experience and Results

22. Shulman CM (1977) Method of a combined surgical treatment of compressive forms of lumbar osteochondrosis with alloplastic material of the damaged intervertebral discs. Vopr Neirokhiv 2: 17–23 (in Russian)
23. Van Steenburgghe MH (1956) Perfectionnements aux prothèses articulaires. FR–PS 1.122.034, 28.5.1956
24. Substad JA (1972) Prothese zum Ersatz einer beschädigten oder degenerierten Bandscheibe und Verfahren zu ihrer Herstellung. DE-AS 2.203.242, 24.1.1972
25. Wittig Ch, Müller RT, Staudte HW, Behrens K (1989) Bandscheibenprothese SB Charité – Erfolge und Mißerfolge anhand von Frühergebnissen. Med Orthop Tech 109: 70–74

Development of a Functional Disc Spacer (Artificial Disc)

C.K. Lee[1], N.A. Langrana[2], J.R. Parsons[1] and M.C. Zimmerman[1]

There are basically two different types of prostheses; replacement of the nucleus pulposus alone and subtotal or total replacement of the intervertebral disc. Preliminary results of research on an "artificial disc" which has adequate compression and compression-torsion properties and can be manufactured with biocompatible materials using either thermoset elastomers with fiber reinforcement or composite thermoplastic elastomers.

Typically, reconstruction for spinal column disorders has been limited to spinal fusion. Recently, investigators in several centers around the world have been developing alternative approaches. These include use of a prosthetic component for the correction of structural or functional deficits of the spinal column while maintaining normal or near normal physiological function of the spinal column, bone, and disc.

Historical Review and Current State of the Art

In recent years, several researchers have investigated artificial devices to partially or totally replace symptomatic and dysfunctional discs. Conceptually, such devices would relieve symptoms while maintaining the functions of the disc – mobility, stability, and weight-bearing. If such a device were available, it could provide similar or more successful long-term results compared to the fusion procedure.

Various types of functional intervertebral endoprostheses have been used or are under investigation. In general, there are two types of prostheses: (1) those involving replacement of the nucleus pulposus alone and (2) those involving total or subtotal replacement of the disc.

Replacement of the Nucleus Pulposus

A spherical metal ball spacer developed by Fernstrom (4) was probably the first endoprosthesis used clinically. The majority of patients, followed up

---

[1] Orthopaedic Surgery, UMDNJ-New Jersey Medical School, 185 South Orange Avenue, Newark, NJ 07103, USA

[2] Mechanical Engineering, Rutgers University, New Brunswick, NJ 08903, USA

The Artificial Disc
Ed. by M. Brock, H.M. Mayer and K. Weigel
© Springer-Verlag Berlin Heidelberg 1991

from 4 to 7 years, showed collapse of the disc space due to migration of the metal ball into the vertebral body. Other researchers (2, 5) have suggested silicone fluids contained in a plastic tube or a silicone rubber nucleus to replace the nucleus pulposus. Recently, Ray [10] described a more sophisticated design for nuclear replacement. The device is made of two, fluid-filled, semipermeable tubes. No report of clinical trials or basic biomechanical information on the device is available to date.

Total or Subtotal Replacement of the Intervertebral Disc

This type of prosthesis requires removal of the nucleus pulposus and partial or total removal of the annulus fibrosus. Several different devices have been tested in a limited number of patients or are being investigated in in vitro studies:

1. *Low friction sliding surfaces*: Design by Hoogland and associates [6]; Limited clinical trials of Link intervertebral endoprosthesis SB Charite.
2. *Spring system*: Design by Patil [9]; no detailed information on mechanical properties or in vitro or in vivo test results available.
3. *Fluid-filled elastic chamber contained in metal cup endplates*: Design by Froning [5]; no information is available about mechanical characteristics of the device.
4. *Elastic disc prosthesis made of rubber or other bioelastomers*: Design by Stubstad and associates [12, 13]; silicone-Dacron prosthesis – animal study and mechanical study showed some initial promising results; however, long term results were not as successful. Steffee's [11] device has been tried in a limited number of patients with early encouraging results.
   The authors of this paper have been engaged in research activities for designing and testing various disc prostheses in our orthopaedic laboratory.

Development of a Functional Disc Spacer (Artificial Disc) at the New Jersey Medical School

This project has been conducted in collaboration with Rutgers University Department of Mechanical Engineering and Johnson and Johnson Orthopaedic Research in New Jersey.

During the past several years, research activities for designing and testing various disc prostheses have been conducted in the authors' laboratories. The first phases of the research included: (1) identification of biocompatible materials which have suitable biomechanical properties; (2) design and fabrication of a prototype disc for mechanical parametric studies; (3) finite element analysis of the prosthetic disc; (4) mechanical testing of various disc prosthesis designs. The next phase of the research was the in vitro testing of disc prostheses after implantation in human cadaveric spines. The last two phases of the research were: (1) studies on the attachment of the disc material to bone (in vivo rabbit study) (2) histological and mechanical studies of in vivo disc replacement in the canine lumbar spine. The bone attachment study (rabbits) was recently published [1] and indicated that appropriately incorporated hydroxyapatite particles on the surface of a thermoplastic elastomer implant provide very satisfactory bony attachment by bone ingrowth and direct attachment mechanisms. The in vivo canine study is underway.

Three different biomaterials were studied: silicone rubber with and without Dacron fiber reinforcement, polyurethane with and without fiber reinforcement, and C-Flex (Concept Polymer Technologies Inc., Clearwater, FL USA) without fiber reinforcement.

The results of mechanical tests demonstrated that silicone rubber discs with or without fiber reinforcement were found to be unsuitable for artificial discs. This is contrary to the results published by Urbaniak et al. [13] Structural rigidity and mechanical strength of silicone Dacron composite discs were far below the lower normal limit of the natural disc.

An artificial disc which has the appropriate mechanical properties (compared to the natural disc) could be manufactured by using the following material and design techniques which are based on theoretical analyses:

1. *Multicomponent thermoplastic design*: The design consists of a central core (nucleus) of relatively soft polymer contained by a more rigid polymer annulus with still more rigid end plates (Fig. 1). The relative areas of the

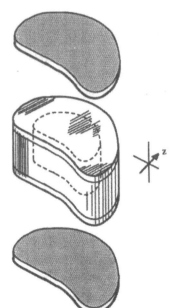

Fig. 1. Thermoplastic elastomeric disc spacer. Three different durometers: nucleus, annulus, and endplates

annulus and nucleus can be adjusted to provide an appropriate overall mechanical response to axial compression. The torsional response of the device was adjusted by changing the rigidity of the annulus. The thermoplastic material used in this design is C-Flex, a polysiloxane-modified, styrene-ethylene/butylene-styrene block copolymer.

2. Fiber-reinforced thermoset design: This design consists of three components analogous to the natural end plates, annulus, and nucleus. In order to obtain the desired mechanical properties of the disc, a variety of material properties for each component were examined. In particular, fiber-reinforced constructions were evaluated for the prosthetic annulus to mimic the normal anatomy. These constructions consisted of multiple layers of fibers with each layer having a uniform orientation to the circumference of the disc. The variables examined in the present study included: (a) orientation of the fiber layers 0°, +45°, and −45°; (b) number of fiber layers; (c) order of the reinforcing layers. The materials used in the manufacturing of these prostheses consisted of a commercially available, two part polyurethane elastomer which is provided in three different grades, each grade having a different durometer (Shore). A40 is the least hard, with an intermediate Shore, A70 and A100 being the hardest. Dacron fibers were used throughout for the reinforcing layers.

The results of mechanical tests of the fiber-reinforced discs indicated that the addition of three and four layers of (0°/+45°/−45°) prepreg fiber-reinforced material in the annular region resulted in the doubling of axial stiffness; torsional stiffness increased by a factor of two to four relative to unreinforced discs. The increase in mechanical properties demonstrated the need for reinforcement in this design. The results further demonstrated that, properly developed, this design exhibited properties similar to those of the natural disc.

The above two artificial disc prostheses (thermoplastic and thermoset biomaterials) have mechanical properties similar to the natural disc and hence may be tolerated better and provide better function than others.

General Considerations

All of the above devices for reconstruction of the disc have been developed for restoration of the structural and functional integrity of the column to a state as close as possible to normal.

Devices for this purpose are considered "long–term" or "permanent" implants and require many important standards including but not limited to the following:

1. Materials to be used must be biocompatible; causing no untoward local tissue reaction, such as inflammatory or foreign body reaction, nor any untoward systemic effects, such as carcinogenicity or organ toxicity.

Materials should also have appropriate mechanical strength under various loading conditions.

2. Design and manufacturing processes should be reliable and reproducible for desired structure and function of the implant. The final device should not be contaminated by any hazardous materials absorbed during the manufacturing process. The final device should be able to withstand an acceptable sterilization procedure without alteration of the material or design characteristics.

3. The operative procedure for the replacement with the device should be relatively easy and safe with little or no serious complications.

4. A device implanted in vivo should have short- and long-term stability and function.

The in vivo stability of the device is usually determined by characteristics of the materials used, design and function of the device, and operative procedure. The greatest concern regarding implantable devices is in vivo fixation or attachment. Mechanical fixation using nails, hooks, screws, staples, etc. are usually considered temporary fixation methods. For permanent fixation, bone ingrowth or cementing techniques have been in use for various orthopaedic and dental procedures. Permanent fixation by means of bone ingrowth has been under intense investigation. Most results suggest that attachment to cancellous bone is extremely difficult, as with the tibial plateau and acetabulum implants. For these areas, metal-backed plastic implants with cement fixation seem to provide the most reliable fixation.

Another method of obtaining in vivo implant stability is a mechanical interlocking between the host bone and the device, as in the cup arthroplasty or Austin Moore prosthesis in the femoral canal. The tissue reaction at the interface is usually affected by the material's tissue biocompatibility and mechanical compatibility between the device and the surrounding bone.

The in vivo stability of implants is also affected by any change in material characteristics due to long-term exposure to the in vivo environment.

Development of successful devices for replacement/reconstruction of the disc and/or vertebral column is in its infancy, but it is a noble idea and a worthwhile pursuit.

References

1. Boone PS, Zimmerman MC, Gutteling E, Lee CK, Parsons JR, Langrana NA (1989) Applied biomaterials J Biomed Mater Res 23: 183–199
2. Edeland HG (1985) Some additional suggestions for an intervertebral disc prosthesis. J Biomed Eng 7: 57–62
3. Fassio B, Ginestie JF (1978) Prosthese discale en silicone. Etude experimentale et premieres observations cliniques. Nouv Presse Med 21: 207
4. Fernstrom U (1966) Arthoplasty with intercorporal endoprosthesis in herniated disc and in painful disc. Acta Chir Scand Suppl 355: 154–159
5. Froming N (1974) Artificial intervertebral disc. United States Patent file

6. Hoogland T, Steffee AD, Black JD, Greenwald AS (1978) Total lumbar intervertebral disc replacement: Testing of a new articulating spacer in human cadaver spines. Transactions of the 24th Orthopaedic Research Society Meeting. Feb. 21–23
7. The Link intervertebral endoprosthesis SB Charite by Waldemar Link (GmbH Co) Barkhausenweg 10, 2000 Hamburg 63 FRG
8. Main JA, Wells ME, Strauss AM (1987) Dynamic vertebral body replacement: A proposed prosthetic device. Presented at the Winter Annual Meeting of the Am Soc of Mech Engineers Boston, Mass, Dec 13–18
9. Patil AA (1982) Artificial intervertebral disc. United States Patent file
10. Ray CD (1988) Artificial Disc, presented at the Challenge of the Lumbar Spine '88 Meeting, San Antonio, Texas, Nov. 9–13
11. Steffee A (1988) Artificial disc. Presented at the Challenge of the Lumbar Spine '88 Meeting, San Antonio, Texas, Nov. 9–13
12. Stubstad JA, Urbaniak JR, Kahn P (1975) Prosthesis for Spinal Repair. United States Patent file
13. Urbaniak JR, Bright DB, Hopkins JR (1973) Replacement of intervertebral discs in chimpanzees by silicone–dacron implants: A preliminary report. J Biomat Res Symposium. 4: 165–186

The Triazine Carbon Fiber-Reinforced Disc Prosthesis: Biomechanical and Biological Properties

J. HARMS and H. BÖHM

Introduction

Each year, 40000–50000 disc operations are performed in the Federal Republic of Germany; thus, the disc is the part of the vertebral column most strongly exposed to wear. Unsatisfactory results are obtained in about 10% of disc operations necessitating further therapy. Some of the failures are surely due to instability of the motion segment as a result of discectomy. This applies particularly to patients whose operations also involve creation of lesions in the dorsal structures (partial resection of the joint facets).

Apart from iatrogenic damage to stability of the motion segment, there are, however, also loosenings caused by disc degeneration without herniation. These are manifested in gaping of the disc or in retrolisthesis. Importance must also be attached to rotatory instability, radiological detection of which is, however, difficult. Instability of the motion segment generally leads to lower back pain, treated by relief measures – physiotherapy, orthesis, or surgery.

If surgical fixation is performed as a result of instability of the motion segment, both the patient and the physician must be aware of the fact that this is an unphysiological intervention. A motion segment is eliminated from the chain of the vertebral column, which leads to an interruption of the otherwise harmonious movement sequence of the vertebral column as a whole. Blockage of a segment can, in turn, be the cause of lower back pain; however, this is usually less severe than the complaints induced by instability.

The sometimes unsatisfactory results following stabilizing procedures explain the long-standing desire to obviate this intervention by finding a disc replacement that at least partially preserves the flexibility of the affected motion segment.

Basic Considerations Concerning Disc Replacement

Construction of an artificial disc must be preceded by precise analysis of the original and of the adjacent vertebrae.

Rehabilitationskrankenhaus Karlsbad-Langensteinbach, W-7516 Karlsbad, FRG

The Artificial Disc
Ed. by M. Brock, H.M. Mayer and K. Weigel
© Springer-Verlag Berlin Heidelberg 1991

Regarded in a purely mechanistic sense, the vertebral column consists of at least two mobile columns: an anterior one comprising the vertebral bodies and the interjacent vertebral disc, and a posterior one composed of the bilateral rows of joints. When bending forward or backward, these two columns move in opposite directions, i.e., the vertebral column, when compressed in the front, is drawn apart at the back and vice versa. This permits the vertebral column to move freely without damaging neural structures.

The connection of two vertebral bodies via a disc was designated by Junghans as a semijoint, since the actual characteristics of a joint are absent. Mobility in the anterior column is rendered possible by a corresponding deformation of the disc, which resumes its original shape again after completion of the movement. This mobility is achieved by elastic deformation of the nucleus pulposus and the anulus fibrosus. It must also be kept in mind that deformation of the disc is determined by the geometry of the vertebral joints, i.e., the vertebral joints themselves permit movement only to a certain degree. This means that regular disc function depends on the intactness of the dorsal joints. The angular mobility of the individual motion segment in the lumbar region ranges between 6° and 8°. In addition to this mobility function, the disc also acts as an axial load buffer. We therefore consider it necessary for a successful disc prosthesis to satisfy three requirements:

1. The joint mechanics of the dorsal vertebral joints must remain undisturbed.
2. The disc prosthesis must permit angular mobility of the motion segment by an adjusted alteration in the axes of rotation.
3. The disc prosthesis must also be able to take over the buffer function of the normal disc.

Construction of the TCF Disc

Based on these considerations, we constructed a disc composed of two, carbon fiber-reinforced, triazine resin (TCF) plates encasing an elastomer core of silicone rubber. This disc prosthesis thus represents a "bumper" with limited mobility. Similar constructions are also used as buffering elements in bridges. Due to the different shapes of the lumbar intervertebral spaces, we worked with two models (Fig. 1). The TCF plates are aligned either in a plane-parallel manner or at an angle to each other. The latter model is intended particularly for the segment L5/S1. The "outer" surface of the TCFT plates, which comes into contact with bone, is convex and coated with bioactive hydroxyapatite.

TCF is an implant material developed by Bosch and based on thermoset plastics strengthened by carbon fibers. The thermoset plastic matrix is triazine resin, which has proven to be very biocompatible in numerous animal and cell culture investigations. The term "biocompatible" signifies here that the TCF

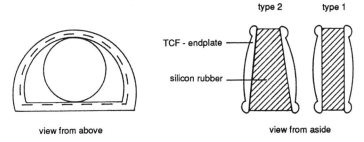

Fig. 1. Sandwich-like construction of the disc prosthesis: TCF end plates and silicone rubber core. Note the two different shapes corresponding to the different geometries of the disc cavities. Convex end plates improve the configuration

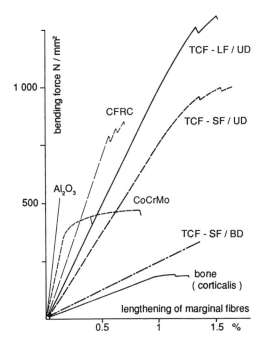

Fig. 2. Strength curves comparing bone, cobalt-based alloy, aluminum oxide ceramic, and TCF. Different arrangements of the carbon fibers: KF = short fiber, LF = long fiber, UD = unidirectional, BD = bidirectional

resin neither produces undesirable tissue reactions nor is attacked by body fluids.

Mechanical Properties of TCF

Mechanical Strength

The stress-strain curves (Fig. 2) show the range of variation of the physical properties of TCF. For comparison, the strength characteristics have been plotted for bone, a cobalt-based alloy, and Al_2O_3 ceramic. The mechanical properties of TCF can be adjusted not only to those of bone, but also to those of metal or ceramic. However, the specific gravity of TCF is considerably lower than that of the latter materials. Different values for the mechanical strength of TCF can be achieved by varying the content of the reinforcing fibers, by utilizing long or short fibers, and by varying the orientation of such fibers.

Dynamic Strength

In Figure 3, the vibration strength curves have been plotted for two TCF discs of differing rigidity and compared with the vibration strength curve of a metallic endoprosthesis made of a cobalt-chromium-molybdenum alloy. Component parts made of TCF clearly reach or surpass the dynamic strength of the cobalt–chromium–molybdenum alloy.

Creep Behavior of TCF

The creep behavior of a material under loading conditions is a measure of its shape stability and thus an indicator of whether relative displacements can occur between bone and implant. Figure 4 was derived from developmental work on the construction of artificial acetabula. The deformation behavior of polyethylene and TCF acetabula embedded in bone cement was demonstrated in a joint simulation test. In the case of TCF, no further deformation was observed after an initial displacement caused by the bone cement setting in the holder. The polyethylene acetabulum, on the other hand, showed strong creeping throughout the entire course of the experiment. Such displacement can endanger the desired direct contact with bone and thus lead to loosening of the bone-implant contact.

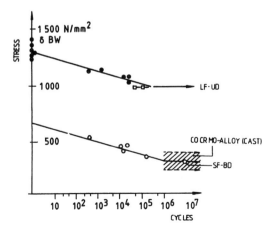

Fig. 3. Repeated bending-stress strength of TCF (SF = short fiber, LF = long fiber, UD = unidirectional, BD = bidirectional) and cobalt-chromium-molybdenum

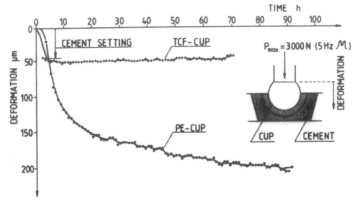

Fig. 4. Creep behavior of acetabula of TCF and polyethylene (*PE*)

Buffering Properties of TCF

The buffering properties of implant materials are important criteria in the construction of endoprostheses. From the viewpoint of buffer function, these properties seem to be even more important in the construction of disc prostheses than in that of hip endoprostheses. Good buffering means that shock-determined vibrations are transmitted to the bone to only a very limited extent.

The buffering (damping) values for TCF and other implant materials are presented in Table 1. TCF has nearly the same high buffering values as polyethylene; those for metal and ceramic are markedly lower. This means that vibrations or shocks are absorbed much better by TCF implants than by metal or ceramic implants. Thus, relative displacement between bone and implant can be largely avoided. The mechanical properties of TCF can be summarized as follows:

Table 1. Elasticity behavior of various implant materials SF = short fiber; LF = long fiber; UD = unidirectional; BD = bidirectional

	Density	Fiber content (%)	Flexural strength (N/mm^2)	E modulus (N/mm^2)	Damping
TCF–LF/UD	1.5	50	1200	100000	$50 \cdot 10^{-4}$
TCF–SF/UD	1.5	50	1000	75000	$50 \cdot 10^{-4}$
TCF–SF/BD	1.3	30	250	20000	$50 \cdot 10^{-4}$
	1.4	40	400	30000	$50 \cdot 10^{-4}$
Al$_2$O$_3$	3.9	–	400	380000	$\sim 3 \cdot 10^{-4}$
CoCrMo Cast alloy	8.3	–	800–900	240000	$7 \cdot 10^{-4}$
Polyethylene	0.94	–	30	800	$130 \cdot 10^{-4}$
Bone Corticalis			100–200	10–20000	

1. The strength properties of TCF can be varied to a high degree.
2. The vibration strength of metallic materials can easily be reached or surpassed by TCF.
3. The creep behavior, as an expression of the stability of shape, is much more favorable for TCF than for polyethylene. Mutual displacement at the bone-implant junction can thus be avoided.
4. The vibration buffering of TCF is similar to that of polyethylene. Thus, transmission of shock and vibrations to bone is minimal. In this way, relative displacement between bone and implant can also be reduced.

Biological Properties of TCF

Stability of TCF

Stability tests performed by the Institut für Kunststoffprüfung at the University of Stuttgart revealed a pronounced tendency of polyethylene to degrade. TCF, on the other hand, proved to be completely stable with respect to oxidation and exposure to reducing agents. Tests on the effects of elevated temperatures for a period of 10000 likewise showed no relevant alterations in TCF that would limit its application as an implant material.

Biological Properties of TCF Based on Animal Studies

Dogs were implanted with artificial hip joints, the acetabulum consisting of TCF, and the femur head of ceramic. The following findings were obtained:

1. . *Capsular Regeneration.* This showed a regular structure with a synovia-like inner cell layer (Fig. 5). There was neither granuloma formation nor toxic tissue reaction. The capsular regeneration product displayed particle deposits that varied in size. Some particles consisted of small pieces of carbon fibers, but particles of synthetic material could also be detected. Small particles were stored within macrophages; larger ones were surrounded by foreign body giant cells. Occasional carbon fiber particles could be detected in the para-aortic lymph nodes. These fibers remained nonreactive within the lymph nodes and were usually stored in macrophages.
2. *Bony Reactions.* There was very good adaptation of the bone to the acetabulum (Fig. 6). In the area of the pressure-loaded anchorage sites, the bone was only separated from the prosthesis by a thin connective tissue membrane. In other places there seemed to be a direct bone-implant contact.

When the acetabula was coated with hydroxyapatite, the implant-bone interface was even more favorable. In many areas, there was direct

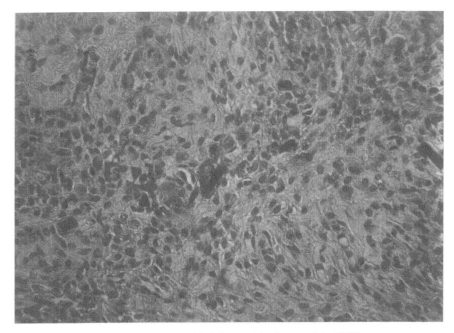

Fig. 5. Pseudocapsule around a dog hip joint prosthesis containing TCF

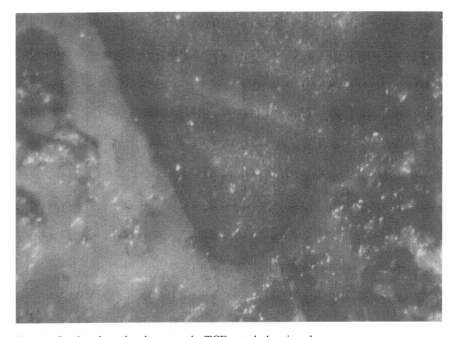

Fig. 6. Implant-bone border around a TCF acetabulum in a dog

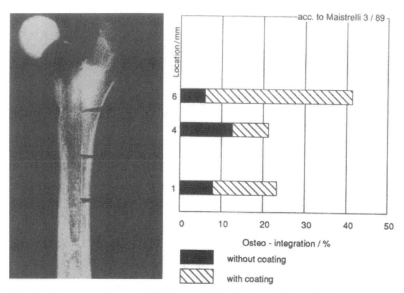

Fig. 7. Bone growth onto TCF femur shafts in dogs. The *solid bars* indicate the bone connection rate as a percentage of that of the uncoated shafts. The corresponding balues for the coated shafts are given by the *shaded bars*

interlocking of bone with the implant surface. A connective tissue membrane could no longer be detected here.

In more recent studies, TCF shafts were implanted in dogs. Both uncoated and hydroxyapatite-coated shafts were used. They were examined to determine to what extent their surface was covered with compact bone. Bone slices were then resected at a precisely defined site an used to determine the bone connection rate.

Figure 7 shows that coating with hydroxyapatite considerably improves the bone connection rate.

Stress Protection with TCF

In these experiments, metallic and TCF shafts were implanted in dogs. After an implantation period of 12 months, the porosity of the bone surrounding the implant was determined.

Porosity can be regarded as a measure of the stress protection offered by an implant. It is clearly recognizable that the bone growing onto a TCF shaft is considerably less porous than that surrounding the cobalt-chromium-molybdenum shaft (Fig. 8). There is practically no difference between a coated and an uncoated TCF shaft.

It can be concluded from these studies that the mechanical properties of TCF are well-adapted to bone substance. Thus, the physiological loading

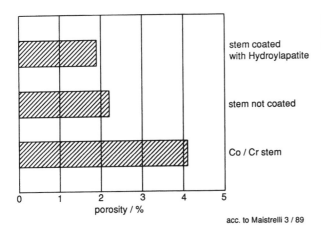

Fig. 8. Stress protection by femur shafts of different materials in the dog

capacity of the bone is largely preserved. The biological properties of TCF can be summarized as follows:

1. TCF is resistant to oxidation and also remains stable in the presence of reducing agents (body fluids).
2. Histological studies reveal good biocompatibility.
3. The use of hydroxyapatite coated TCF results in very good interlocking of bone and implant.
4. Adaptation of TCF to the elasticity modulus of bone prevents a stress protection reaction by the surrounding bone. This can be of decisive importance in the sense of a long-term bone-implant connection.

Connection of TCF Plates with Silicone Rubber

The favorable results with respect to the mechanical properties and biocompatibility of TCF prompted our decision to also use it for the construction of a disc prosthesis.

It has already been mentioned that the artificial disc is composed of two TCF "end plates" firmly connected by an elastomer core of silicone rubber. The permissible angular mobility depends on the thickness of the silicone rubber layer. With a thickness of 9 mm, an angular mobility of +/− 7° is possible, which is regarded as adequate for lumbar segments.

Decisive for prosthesis function is adhesion of the silicone rubber to the TCF plates. Experimental results on this are as follows:

1. *Test of adhesive strength.* The strength of adhesion of silicone rubber to the TCF plates was tested by using the equipment shown in Fig. 9 and measuring the strength necessary to remove a rubber strip fixed to a TCF plate. Figure 10 shows the pull-off strengths of four different samples; the

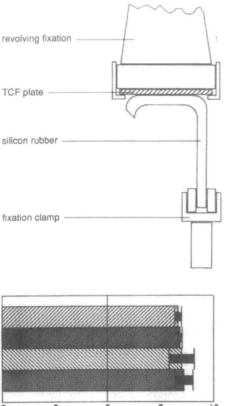

Fig. 9. Experimental setup for testing TCF/silicone adhesion

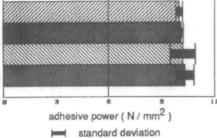

Fig. 10. Adhesive strengths under various production conditions

adhesive strength depends only slightly on the different production conditions. The range of deviation of the adhesive strength is also negligible.

2. *Strength of adhesion of silicone rubber to the TCF plate after continuous loading.* Loading of the prosthesis in the vertebral column was simulated by means of a swiveling tension device on a servohydraulic testing machine (Fig. 11). More than 25 discs have been tested with load reversal swivel cycles between 300000 and 5 million. In these tests, the disc prosthesis was subjected to a constant load of 1 kN. The swivel angle was $+/- 3.5°$. The test was also performed wih a frequency of 5 Hz and under load control, i.e., the basic load was kept approximately constant during the swiveling procedure.

Figure 12 shows the adhesive strengths of two disc prostheses of different thicknesses with their initial loading values or preloaded with 2 million load reversals under the above conditions: No great difference

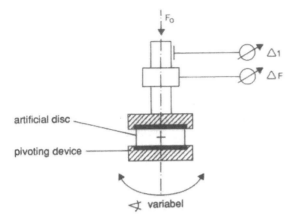

Fig. 11. Experimental setup for testing continuous loading of the TCF disc

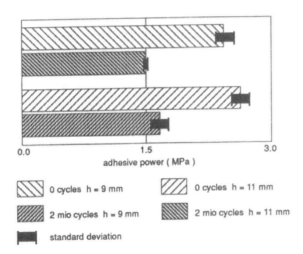

Fig. 12. Influence of vibration strength on adhesive strength. *Broad hatches*, initial loading values; *narrow-hatches*, adhesive strength of prostheses preloaded with 2 million load reversals

was evident between the two discs. Even after 2 million load reversals, the adhesive strength was still great enough not to endanger the function of the disc prosthesis.

3. *Varying tensile stress test.* In the varying tensile stress test, increasing and decreasing distraction tensions were applied to both TCF plates. The forces exerted here ranged between 100 and 1000 N; the tensions were increased and decreased with a frequency of 5 Hz. The TCF/silicone rubber connection proved to be stable in this test as well: With load reversals of more than 5 million, the disc was destroyed by tearing of the rubber but not by loosening of the connection between the TCF plate and

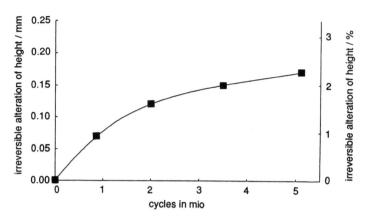

Fig. 13. Irreversible changes in thickness following continuous loading absolute values in millimeters on the *left ordinate* and the changes in percentages on the *right ordinate*

the silicone rubber. In interpreting this test of adhesive strength, it must be considered that the prosthesis is seldom exposed to tensions when implanted in the vertebral column.

4. *Irreversible change in disc thickness after loading.* The decrease in disc thickness under a load of 1000 N with 5 million load reversals is practically negligible (Fig. 13).
5. *Biocompatibility of silicone rubber:* Silicone rubber has long been known for its good biocompatibility. In order to ensure that during production of the disc prostheses no reactions occurred which altered biocompatibility, different prostheses were submitted to cell culture examination. It was thus possible to determine those production conditions under which there was no reaction between the rubber disc and the TCF plates that may have resulted in undesirable biological effects. This ensured that the TCF/silicone rubber connection could be regarded as a biocompatible one.

Summary

The artificial disc described here is composed of two TCF end plates firmly connected by an elastomer core of silicone rubber. This disc represents a buffering element with limited mobility as frequently employed in other fields of technology, e.g., bridge building. TCF was chosen as the implant material for the disc end plates because of its biomechanical and biological suitability. The connection between the TCF end plates and silicone rubber is optimized so as to ensure firm adhesion of the silicone rubber to the end plates. Cell culture experiments have proven that the production process does not cause undesirable changes in biocompatibility.

Subject Index

a-delta fibers 56
acrylonitrile 50
adhesive strength 93
Al2O3 ceramic 88
allergenic effect 15
alloarthroplasty 19
allograft bone 59
alloplastic materials 23–25
aluminium oxide 13, 17
annulus-nucleus loading ratio 48
anterior interbody 65
anulus fibrosus 5, 86
aortic prosthesis 53
arthrodesis 23, 46
articular
– orthogonal theory 5
– prosthesis 1
artificial
– devices 79
– disc (see sep. referral) 1, 2, 23, 70, 79
– hip joints 90
– intervertebral disc prosthesis 24
– joints 1
artificial disc 1, 2, 23, 70, 79
– prostheses 57
– replacement 6–8, 10
autoimmune response 55
autologous bone chips 53
axial stiffness 82

Babgy concept 60
Babgy's baskets 60
back pain 64
ball prosthesis 69
bending-stress strength 88
bioactive glass-ceramic (Ceravital)
  24–26, 33
biocompatibility 82, 93, 96
biocompatible materials 80, 86
Bioglass 24
bioinert implant materials 24
biological properties 90
biomaterials
– thermoplastic 82

– thermoset 82
biomechanical
– compatibility 20
– properties 80
bisegmental disc replacements 74
blind percutaneous access 45
– postero-lateral 45
bone
– allograft 59
– autologous bone chips 53
– cancellous 25
– fresh frozen human 59
– frozen cadaver bone grafts 59
– graft 62
– homograft 47
– homologous bone grafting 23
– ingrowth 83
– reactions 90
– substance 92
buffering properties 89
burr hole 25

c-fibers 56
C-Flex 81, 82
cadaveric testing 70
cage fusions 63
cancellous bone 25
capsular regeneration 90
carbon 24
– fibers 86
carcinogenicity 82
ceramic 48
– implants 89
– materials 17
ceravital 25, 26, 33
cervical
– fusions 24, 60
– vertebral bodies 3
Charite modular 69
chemonucleolysis 39
Chirulen 70
chondrocytes 36, 56
chondrocytic synthesis 56
chondroitin 55

Subject Index

chromium 13–15
cobalt 15
– alloy 19
– cast alloy 19
cobalt-based alloy 17, 88
cobalt-chromalloy (ISO 5832/IV) 70
cobalt-chromium implants 29
cobalt-chromium-molybdenum
– alloy 24, 88
– shaft 92
cobalt-chromium-molybdenum-based cast
 alloy 13
CoCrMo alloys 24, 88
CoCrMo-ASTM-F75 sintered implants 25
"cold-flow" 70
cold formation 19
compatibility
– biocompatibility 93, 96
– biomechanical 20
– mechanical 83
– tissue biocompatibility 83
compressive strength 50
contra indications 74
copolymer 50, 82
corrosion resistance 14
creep behavior 88, 90
CT 64, 65, 74
cylindrical implants 25

Dacron fiber 81
decompression 64
deep-vein thromboses 74
deformation strength 62
disc(s)
– artificial 1, 2, 23, 70, 79
– degeneration (see sep. referral) 74
– disease, lumbar 2
– dysfunctional 79
– endoprosthesis 33, 70
– herniation 36
– intervertebral 3, 54, 69
– lumbar 54
– material 81
– prostheses (see sep. referral) 58, 81, 86
– replaced 1
– replacement(s) (see sep. referral) 6–8,
 10, 74
– replacement surgery 76
– reptured cervical 23
– spacer, functional 79
– substitute 48
– surgery 69
– TCF 86
disc degeneration 74
– monosegmental 74
– oligosegmental 74

disc prostheses 58, 81, 86
– artificial 57
– artificial intervertebral 24
– monosegmental 74
disc replacement(s) 6–8, 10, 74
– artificial 6–8, 10
– bisegmental 74
– monosegmental 74
discectomy 62
discogenic pain, 55 ,56, 64
discography 35, 74
– provocative 64
distance protection 69
disturbed wound healings 74
dynamic behavior 70
dysfunctional discs 79

elastic
– deformation 86
– recoil 62
elasticity 15, 17
end plates 1
endoprosthesis 13, 69, 79, 88
– disc 33, 70
– functional intervertebral 79
– steel ball 69
epiduritis 10
expansion bullet 47
extraperitoneal route 70

facet joints 46, 69, 74, 76
– screening injections 64
– subluxation 70
facetectomy 63
"failed backs" 74
fatigue
– fractures 75
– strength 17, 19
Fernström's ball prostheses 69
fibers, a-delta 56
flavum ligaments 62, 63
flexibility 15, 16
flexible silicon plastics 69
"floating" fusion 64
foreign body reaction 48, 82
fracture(s) 17
– fatigue 75
– implant 76
– prosthetic shaft 17
– stress 75
– vertebral 10
– of vertebral body end plates 70
fresh frozen human bone 59
frozen-dried cadaver bone grafts 59
functional
– disc spacer 79

Subject Index

99

- intervertebral endoprostheses 79
fusion(s) 8
- cage 63
- cervical 24, 60
- "floating" 64
- interbody 46, 53, 59, 65
- lumbar interbody 60
- posterior lumbar interbody fusions (PLIF) 60
- secondary 75
- spinal 79
- threaded fusion cages 63, 64

gene technology 20
Giemsa solution 26
glass-ceramics (Ceravital) 24–26, 32, 33
glycolic acid 20
graft bone 62
granuloma formation 90

HAC coated screw dowels 48
Hastings approach 45
hip joint
- shafts 13
- sockets 13
histomorphometry 24, 30
homograft bone 47
homologous bone grafting 23
Hook's rule 16
hot formation 19
hyaluronic acid 53, 55
hydrogels 50
hydrophilic
- gels 49
- jells 50
hydroxyapatite 23, 24, 86, 90, 93
- ceramic slurry 47
- formulations 60
hydroxyehtylmethacrylate 49
hygroscopic hyaluronic acid 53
hyperlordosis 3, 4
hypersensitivity reactions 15
hysrosyapatite particles 81
hysteresis 70

iliac spine, posterior 62
implant(s)
- ceramic 89
- cobalt-chromium 29
- CoCrMo-ASTM-F75 sintered 25
- cylindrical 25
- fractures 76
- intradiscal 35, 47
- metal 89
- metal-backed plastic 83
- migrations 76

- osteosyntheses 13, 16, 17
- plate 65
- smooth surfaced titanium 33
- thermoplastic elastomer 81
implant titanium 15
- alloy monolayer sintered 30
- alloy sintered 25
- mesh 23
instability, painful 69
interbody, anterior 65
interbody fusion(s) 46, 53, 59, 65
- lumbar 60
- posterior lumbar 60
interfacial load transmission 24
interspinous ligaments 63
intervertebral
- disc(s) 3, 54, 69
- foramen/foramina 6, 10, 69, 75
- space 69
intradiscal
- implant(s) 35, 47
- polymerization 39
- prostheses 53
intranuclear pressure 55
irreversible change 96

joint balls 13
joint mechanics 86

keratin sulphate 55
kinetic center 69

lactic acid 20
laminotomy 62
latent spinal infections 74
lateral
- recess 38, 46
- stenosis 64
leg pain 64
ligamenta flava 5
link prosthesis 39
long-term stability 83
lumbar
- disc disease 2, 54
- interbody fusions 60
- kyphosis 3
- spine 3
lumbosacral
- angle 3
- biodynamics 10
- junction 54
- lordosis 3

material(s)
- alloplastic 23–25
- biocompatible 80

100 Subject Index

material(s), bioinert implant 24
- ceramic 17
- disc 81
- silastic 48
mechanical
- compatibility 83
- fixation 83
memory
- effect 20
- pain 74
metal
- implants 89
- spongiosa 23
metal-backed plastic implants 83
methacrylate 50
methylmethacrylate cement 23
MIF (minimal intervention fenestration)
  45
migration of vertebral body end plates 70
minimal intervention fenestration (MIF)
  45
- percutaneous posterior 45
- postero-medial 45
mobility 79
monosegmental disc
- degeneration 74
- replacements 74
MRI 74
MRL 65
mucopolysaccharide content 54
myelography 74

neural
- structures 86
- tissues 62
neuromeningeal dynamics 9
Ni-Ti memory alloy 23
nickel 13, 15
nickel-titanium (Ni-Ti) 20
niobium 13
non-metal cages 65
normal motion 69
notch tear strength 50
nucleotomy 35, 39
nucleus pulposus 1, 5, 79, 86
nylon 50

oligosegmental disc degeneration 74
oral implantology 24
organ toxicity 82
"osseointegration" 24
osteoarthrosis 74
osteocytes 33
osteoporosis 74
osteoporotic changes 74
osteosyntheses 13, 20

- implant(s) 13, 16, 17
oxidation 93

pain
- back 64
- discogenic 55, 56, 64
- leg 64
- memory 74
pain sense 56
painful instability 69
Palacos 14, 23, 25, 30
PE (see also polyethylene) 13, 19, 89, 90
pedicle screw 65
pediculotomy 63
permanent fixation 83
plate implants 65
PLIF technique 61
PMMA (polymethyl methacrylate) 14,
  23, 25, 30
polyamide pulposus 50
polyester 13, 19
- fibre 50
polyethylene (PE) 13, 19, 89, 90
- acetabulum 88
- (Chirulen) 70
- core 70
- lens core 71
polyglycolic acid 58
polymerization, intradiscal 39
polymers 24
polymethyl methacrylate (PMMA) 14,
  23, 25, 30
- cement (Palacos) 14, 23, 25, 30
polyoxymethylene 14, 19
polytetrafluorethylene (PTFE) (Proplast)
  14, 26, 31
polyurethane(s) 14, 39, 81
- elastomer(s) 40, 82
porosity 91
posterior
- approach 69
- iliac spine 62
- ligaments 62
- longitudinal ligament 5, 36
- lumbar interbody fusions (PLIF) 60
- MIF approach 48
posterolateral percutaneous approach 39,
  43
posteromedial MIF 45
Proplast 14, 26, 31
prosthesis/prostheses
- aortic 53
- articular 1
- artificial disc 57
- artificial intervertebral disc 24
- ball 69

Subject Index

– disc 58, 81, 86
– Fernström's ball 69
– intradiscal 53
– link 39
– silicon-Dacron 80
prosthetic
– joints 58
– nuclei/nucleus 53, 62
– shaft 16
– shaft fractures 17
proteoglycans 55, 56
provocative discography 64
PTFE (Proplast) 14, 26, 31
pure titanium (Contimet) 25, 26

recess, lateral 38, 46
replaced discs 1
replacement 79
replica 1
retrolisthesis 85
rigidity 15, 17
rotatory instability 85
ruptured cervical disc 23

scanning electron microscopy 24, 33
Schmorl "dome" 63
sciatica 35
scoliosis 3, 20
screw dowels, HAC coated 48
secondary fusion 75
semicircular
– hemilaminotomy 63
– laminotomy 62, 63
servohydraulic
– test rig 70
– testing machine 94
shear strength 24
shock absorption 69
shock-determined vibrations 89
shortened intradiscal bullet 48
silastic materials 48
silicon-Dacron prosthesis 80
silicon rubber 14, 81, 93, 96
– nucleus 80
silver 13
smooth surfaced titanium implants 33
spherical metal ball 79
spinal
– column 79
– fusion 79
– infections, latent 74
– segment 69
– surgery 2
spinous process 63
spondylolisthesis 74
spongiosae 62

stability 79, 90
stabilizing procedures 85
stainless steel 17
static testing 70
steel ball endoprostheses 69
strength
– adhesive 93
– bending-stress 88
– compressive 50
– deformation 62
– fatigue 17, 19
– notch tear 50
– shear 24
– tensile 17, 24, 33, 50
– vibration 90
stress
– fractures 75
– protection reaction 93
stress-shielding phenomena 33
stress-strain curves 87
styrene 50
surface roughness 24
surgical instruments 65
swivel(ling)
– angel 94
– procedure 94
synthetic CaPo4 ceramics 24

tantalum 13
TCF
– disc 86
– end plates 96
– plates 86, 93
teflon 19
temperature sense 56
temporary fixation 83
tensile
– strength 17, 24, 33, 50
– stress test 95
thermoplastic biomaterials 82
thermoplastic elastomer(s) 79
– implant 81
thermoset
– biomaterials 82
– elastomers 79
– plastic matrix 86
thixotropic agent 53
threaded
– cages 61
– fusion cages 63, 64
three-column
– concept 4
– spine concept 4
Ti5A12.5Fe alloy 27, 33
Ti6A14V alloy 26, 33
Ti6A14V-slot pattern 27

Ti6A14V-wafer pattern 27
tissue
– biocompatibility 83
– tolerance 14, 20
titanium 13, 14, 17, 24, 48, 53, 61
– alloys (see sep. referral) 24, 25, 30
– cage 62
– (Contimet) 25, 26
– implants 15
– mesh implants 23
titanium alloys 24
– monolayer sintered implants 30
– sintered implants 25
– glass-ceramic composite
   (HIP-titanium-Ceravital) 25
torsional stiffness 82
total hip arthroplasty 24
triazine resin 86

urinary infections 74

vein thromboses, deep 74
vertebral

– ankylosis 23
– body end plates 70, 73
– body infractions 75
– destruction 70
– end plates 55
– fracture 10
vibration
– buffering 90
– strength 90
– strength curves 88

"wobbler" syndrome 60
Wöhler diagram 17, 18

X-ray identification 70

Young's
– elasticity modulus 16
– module 40–42

zirconium 13
zirconium oxide 17
zygapophyseal joints 6, 7

J. M. Cotler, Thomas Jefferson University, Philadelphia, PA;
H. B. Cotler, University of Texas, Houston, TX (Eds.)

Spinal Fusion

Science and Technique

Foreword by A. F. DePalma

1990. XVI, 407 pp. 317 figs. in 570 parts. Hardcover DM 490,–
ISBN 3-540-97054-1

Contents: The Science of Spinal Fusions. – Indications for Spinal Fusion. – Anatomy and Surgical Approaches. – Fusion Techniques. – Postoperative Management. – The Future. – Index.

This thorough volume puts the experience of top professionals into your own hands. The editors and their impressive group of contributors, including researchers, educators, and clinicians, have joined together to bring you this concise, comprehensive reference. Sections relating to history, basic science, surgical indications and techniques, complications, and postoperative management, as well as a philosophical chapter on the future of spine surgery are presented. With the help of over 300 superb illustrations, **Spinal Fusion: Science and Technique** contains the most current and authoritative compilation of knowledge relating to surgical management of disorders of the spine. It will become an essential tool in your working library.

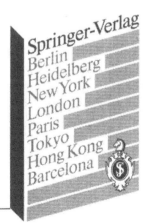

M. Samii, Hannover (Ed.)

Peripheral Nerve Lesions

1990. XVII, 465 pp. 225 figs. 64 tabs.
Hardcover DM 278,- ISBN 3-540-52432-0

This book gives a multidisciplinary and complete summary of the state of the art of peripheral nerve lesions. The chapters cover all aspects of the subject, from experimental research to clinical and surgical topics. Leading international experts describe their experiences and views. The reader is given an up-to-date report based on the newest available information on this subject.

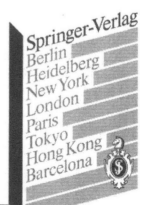

Springer-Verlag
Berlin
Heidelberg
New York
London
Paris
Tokyo
Hong Kong
Barcelona

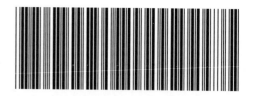